**Good
Health...
Naturally!**

Good Health... Naturally!

20 Steps to Better Nutrition Using Natural Foods

Linda Alger, Priscilla Sanders

International Standard Book Number
0-88290-217-2

Library of Congress Catalog Card Number
83-80405

Horizon Publishers Catalog and Order Number
4025

Printed and Distributed in the
United States of America
by

Horizon
Publishers &
Distributors, Inc.

———————————

50 South 500 West
P.O. Box 490
Bountiful, Utah 84010

Disclaimer

This book is not intended to replace the services of a physician. All matters regarding your health require medical supervision. The ideas expressed by the authors in this book are their own practices gleaned from the study of many other theories.

Acknowledgments

We would like to acknowledge with love and appreciation all those who have helped and inspired us to write this book. Our husbands, Dennis Alger and Jim Sanders, have lent constant support for which we are grateful. We love our children Arlene, Bryan, Christie, David, Elizabeth, and Gregory Alger, and John, Mark, Deidrean, Michael, and Stephen Sanders. We thank them for cheerfully trying our recipes and new foods. We are also grateful to our mothers, Esther N. Boekweg and Macky Grief, who have encouraged us to seek after truth.

Many thanks to Judith Roberson, Sally Hildebrandt, and Jeanne Jensen for proof-reading. We express our thanks to Johanna Hall, of Virginia Beach, Virginia, who continues to teach principles of good nutrition. Iris Syndergaard was of great assistance in the final editing of the book. Also, our thanks go to those mothers who shared examples and experiences. Most important, we would like to acknowledge our Heavenly Father who has inspired and allowed us this opportunity to share our thoughts and ideas with others.

Contents

Introducing
Good Health ... Naturally!

Good Health ... Naturally! features hidden treasures relevant to better nutrition for the mother and her family. Through the ages, man has been admonished to practice sound principles of nutrition. Encouragement has been given by various organizations to acquire appropriate skills in food selection and preparation. This book will help to achieve these goals.

The purpose of this book is not only to show the whys of improved nutrition, but how to apply these ideas. First, the aspects of personal awareness are highlighted. Next, surprising truths about refined and processed foods are explained. The Twenty Steps to Better Nutrition include food choices and methods of preparing such nutritious foods as homemade yogurt, buttermilk, salad dressings, and whole-wheat bread. Also discussed are ways to avoid junk foods. We, the authors, have applied these steps in our own lives and we have reaped the results of exceptional health.

To make reaching each step fun and challenging, a goal-selection sheet has been provided to be filled in by the reader as each step is mastered. Sections on menu planning, baking day tips, grocery shopping guidelines, ways to stretch the food dollar, food storage ideas, and sample recipes are also included to help with the transition to better nutrition. This practical handbook, kitchen tested by the authors, would be a valued asset to every homemaker.

Unit 1
Nutritional Awareness

Chapter 1

Beginnings Of Personal Awareness

If you have lost your health temporarily and then had it restored, you know what a blessing good health is. We can do God's work when we enjoy good health. When you have your health, you are truly wealthy. Health is a treasure.

As we understand the principles of good nutrition, we become truly wise. Wisdom can then be used in applying these principles. Health and strength are blessings from the Lord, but we must do our part to keep these treasures.

Priscilla's Story

My interest in better nutrition began a number of years ago. My family and I began to make gradual changes in our eating habits. More whole-wheat bread was eaten; fewer prepackaged cereals.

As I had the opportunity to study more about nutrition, the desire grew within me to help others apply what I had learned. My convictions were growing stronger because I had tested the principles. My family was reaping the benefits of better nutrition through improved health.

So many friends questioned—How do I apply these principles? Where do I begin? How can we ever make so many changes? I had a strong desire to help others experience what I had found to be so beneficial.

Linda and I formulated a plan, taken from our own experiences, to help others apply these ideas on nutrition. This is an action book. The ideas must be applied and tested to see what works for you and your family.

Linda and I realize that there are many different ideas concerning nutrition. We do not claim to have the only approach. This book was written for beginners in nutrition to help them make the change from empty calorie foods to more nutritious foods. Through continued study, you will find which foods are right for you and your health.

My intent is to share the fortune of good health which I have enjoyed. May you find success.

Linda's Story

Wintertime was getting to be unwelcome at our home. The season brought much disease and sickness which spread among family members. I was dragging myself out of bed in the morning worn out from nursing the sick the night before. It seemed I was either going to or coming from the doctors, picking up a prescription or spooning down medicine every three to four hours. I love my family and seeing them in pain caused me to suffer also. I became frustrated and almost discouraged. Yet I knew that to give up was a cop-out. Deep within myself I knew running away was not the answer to any problem. I would face my problems and find a solution.

One mother, with a large family, told me that her doctor offered her some sound advice. He told her to get up in the morning and plan for someone to stay home sick. This helped her handle the unexpected illnesses that upset her busy schedule.

I was unable to settle for this if I could find a better way. I felt I would be coping with the symptoms of the problem (sick family members) and not the problem itself (what made them sick). So I asked myself two questions: (1) What might be the cause of these illnesses? (2) What can I do about them?

In the spring of 1978, I met a lady who offered answers to these questions. I experimented with her advice. As a result, the next three winters came and went, leaving our family in better health than before.

The solution to my problem has been explained within the covers of this book. The success of exceptional health which my family obtained by practicing these twenty steps to better nutrition, created the desire in me to help other mothers who are searching for ways to have better health within their homes. It is my belief that the ideas and principles contained in this book are true. I invite all to try them for themselves. I am confident you will agree that by achieving your goals on the goal sheet and by using the recipes and menu planning charts you will enjoy improved physical and emotional well-being.

Your family's health can be improved by learning ways to apply principles of good nutrition. Throughout this book, the authors have endeavored to share skills and knowledge of ways to use wholesome foods. Applying these ideas can help to nourish and strengthen the body against diseases, dental cavities, and illness. You will also find a twenty-step program to help you practice sound principles of good nutrition. Techniques are given to help you apply the steps, as well as suggestions for the selection and preparation of nutritious foods. Good nutrition will be made easy. When you discover the simple secrets of improving your family's nutritional habits, thereby improving their health, you and your family can have *Good Health ... Naturally!*

Chapter 2

The Truth About Refined and Processed Foods

The beginning of good health is to become nutritionally aware. Most Americans feel that they are somewhat knowledgeable about nutrition. Yet how aware are you personally about what food processors are doing to your food? For years the American diet has become increasingly processed and refined. How easy it is to go to the grocery store for packaged macaroni and cheese dinners, frozen french fries, instant potatoes or pre-sweetened cereals. Consider a typical American breakfast: "enriched" white bread spread with jelly, artificial-imitation orange drink, margarine, possibly imitation eggs or imitation bacon. Lunch may be a bologna on "enriched" white bread, potato chips, a slice of processed cheese and an imitation fruit drink. These typical meals contain large amounts of refined sugar, white flour, additives and preservatives.

Why are these foods so harmful? For one thing, refined and processed foods consumed in such vast quantities by Americans contain few vitamins and minerals. Yet most of us realize that vitamins and minerals are necessary for a healthy body.

Many refining and processing techniques strip food of its nutritive content. Refining of whole-wheat flour into white flour reduces vitamin and mineral content anywhere from 50 to 98 percent, depending on those involved. Refining removes 27 percent of the protein, 57 percent of the panothenic acid, 60 percent of the calcium, 78 percent of the magnesium, 94 percent of the pyridoxine, 66 percent of the riboflavin, 74 percent of the potassium, 50 percent of the linoleic acid, 97 percent of the thiamine and 76 percent of the iron. Twenty-six essential elements are totally or partially removed from flour. White flour is synthetically "enriched" by replacing only three vitamins: thiamine, riboflavin and niacin. A small amount of iron is replaced. Processed flour is then bleached with chlorine dioxide, a chemical which may prove harmful.

16

If you had twenty-six treasures and someone took them and returned four treasures, would you feel "enriched," or robbed? Yet you are "robbed" every time whole-wheat flour is refined into white flour.

Consider refined sugar as an example of what processors do to your food. When was the last time you read an ingredients label? These labels prove that sugar is a major ingredient in most convenience foods.

Why is sugar bad for you? There are a number of reasons. Sugar is being linked to heart disease and may also contribute to circulatory problems which may cause hypertension. Dr. John Yudkin, at the University of London, reports that a person who consumes four ounces (one-half cup) of sugar a day is five times more likely to develop heart disease than is a person who eats half that amount. Through his studies, Dr. Yudkin concludes that sugar is a main cause of heart disease and diabetes, as well as other disorders.[1]

Would you feed your child seven tablespoons of sugar for a snack? Put seven tablespoons of sugar in a bowl to give you an idea of how much that is. Many mothers give little thought to feeding their children commercially prepared fruit pies, yet each of many fruit pies contains seven tablespoons of sugar. Besides, such pastries contain little, if any, nutrition.

Processed cheese serves as another example of what food processors do to our food. Hard cheeses are mixed together by grinding and heating. Emulsifiers, preservatives, artificial color, artificial flavors, stabilizers, other chemicals and high heat are used to process cheese. And each process affects the nutritional content. The end result is not a quality product.

How many times a year do Americans pour instant potatoes from a box rather than peel the real thing? Potato flakes, pre-cut hash browns, french fries, potato pancakes, potato puffs, potato chips, diced potatoes, potatoes au gratin and frozen baked potatoes are common side-dishes. In processed potatoes the vitamins and minerals have been replaced by synthetic vitamins and minerals: preservatives, emulsifiers, antioxidants, stabilizers and thickeners have been added to ensure a longer shelf life. No convenience should be worth the loss of so much nutrition. When brown rice is polished into white rice, it is stripped of many nutrients. Even though it may be "enriched," much is lost in the process.

Even a purposeful selection of foods from the four basic food groups does not assure a balanced diet. Good foods have necessary

1. Gary Null, The New Vegetarian, p. 274.

nutrition taken away in processing and refining. For instance, you may serve canned or fresh green beans for supper. Even though both come from one of the four basic food groups, there is much difference in their nutritional value.

To ensure that you do get necessary nutrients, changes in shopping habits need to be made. Avoid as many commercial products as possible. If a food has been packaged, processed, added to, emulsified, stabilized, colored, or preserved, it becomes a product that is not desirable. A careful reading of each ingredients label should play an essential part in your selection of foods.

After a shopping trip made to read the labels of grocery items usually bought, you should begin to see the need for a change in your eating habits.

You may wonder where to start. You may feel that so many changes are necessary you don't know *where* to begin. A step-by-step program will help. The following chapters will show exactly *what* changes need to be made. They will help you understand *why* the changes are necessary, and *how* to make these changes gradually.

By planning your new nutrition program with the help of this book, you will increase your knowledge of the importance of good nutrition. Learn to appreciate wholesome grains and fresh fruits and vegetables included in the plan.

An intellectual conviction of nutrition is a basic motivation in the test of true principles. Personal experience brings this to excellence. You may combine your previous experiences and knowledge with steps in this nutrition outline to plan, set and achieve the best possible nutrition in your eating habits. Good, established eating habits can play a vital role in your pursuit of success. Once you have applied the first step and made it a part of your nutrition program, you will be on your way. Twenty-one consecutive steps are required before a habit becomes automatic behavior. Work on one step for a week before applying the next step to help make the first step become a habit. Then go on to the next step while still applying the previous ones. (See Contents, Unit II, Twenty Steps to Better Nutrition.) Chapter 24, Goal Selection, will help you plan your goals. If you make your changes gradual your family will be less apt to rebel against your new program.

These steps were written with an understanding love and with a sincere desire to share with you ideas on how we, the authors, built our own families physically, mentally and spiritually. When your body receives the proper fuel, rest, and exercise, you can more readily accomplish your goals in life. You can be an example for others by the sparkle in your eyes, the shine of your hair and a glow which is the glow of good health.

You cannot force better eating habits on your family. However, as mothers you have the responsibility to buy groceries and prepare meals. Remember that faith, love, prayer, creativity and persistence can help you reach your desired goals for better nutrition.

After you have read and tested these principles, may these truths begin to grow in your heart. They are true! They do work! The principles employ plain old "common sense."

If you follow the steps outlined in this book, your health can improve. Days can be better and happier. Improved nutrition will not prevent all illness or disease, but your body will not be as susceptible to them. There will be many more good days for you because you will feel better.

A doctor alone cannot prevent disease. (Doctors often treat people's illnesses and symptoms with medicine and drugs.) It takes a mother who cares!

Unit II
Twenty Steps
To Better Nutrition

Chapter 3

Step 1
Study Nutrition

Colds, flu, sore throats, headaches, arthritis, sinus infection, eczema, pheumonia, and depression are not present in those who enjoy normal health. The effects of these illnesses and many others have been eliminated or greatly reduced for many people through their use of proper nutrition. Some might rationalize their eating habits by saying, "But my cupboards are full of empty-calorie snacks and processed foods. I cannot just throw them out." Or they will apologize for their family with the statement, "I would like to change, but my family would rebel." Although these reasons may contain some truth, the switching-over process is not as difficult as it sounds.

The following story, as related by Linda Joan Alger, will show how she used effective tools to teach better nutrition:

I became determined to change my selection of foods and eating habits for my family of seven because of a nutrition class I had taken in 1978. I knew they, too, would have to gain a strong understanding of the importance of proper nutrition. My desire had turned into commitment to reach my goal of eating more healthful foods and fewer empty calories.

My family had formed the habit of eating sugar-filled fruit pies, chocolate sweet cakes and squeezable white bread bought at a discount bakery. It was unrealistic to change my family's eating habits and to begin overnight to eat only those foods that were living and vital. I would have to throw out almost everything in my pantry, from potato chips to white sugar. With five children to feed that would be impossible. I would

20

make the changes gradually until my pantry was filled with nutritious items, including fresh bagged potatoes, pure maple syrup and raw sunflower seeds.

While meditating one afternoon, as the children were napping, I got an idea on how I could help my family to progress. The answer flashed into my mind to prepare a lesson on the nutritional ideas I had been taught in the nutrition class. I decided evenings set aside for just our family would be a perfect time to introduce my family to the new discoveries learned in the nutrition class which had been taught by dietitian Johanna Hall of Virginia Beach, Virginia.

Previously, I had experienced continual sickness among my five small children. After coming home from the doctor's office the third time in one week, I said to myself, "If this is what motherhood is all about, I do not want any part of it! To go through this every winter has left me feeling unfulfilled and depressed." I was not very happy. My patience was thin. My nerves were frayed. I was tired in the morning and afternoon and exhausted by night. My bed became my best friend, my escape from reality. My goal was just to get through another day.

I was looking for something or someone to help me. Yet it was not until I was lead to the nutrition class that I found the answers to many of my problems—you are what you eat.

I decided a well-planned night with our family would be a starting place for me to teach. I wanted to experience success. Soon ideas for a theme, a special dinner, and a lesson all came to me.

Theme: Feeding our physical bodies the proper foods so our family will be better prepared to achieve our desired goals.

Special Dinner: Baked fish, tossed salad, deviled eggs, homemade applesauce, and sweet acidopholus milk.

Lesson: Liken our bodies to a car explaining that proper fuel for both is needed if they are to run their best. Prepare two trays of food. Explain what food processors do to the food. Explain, and show, the three different parts of the wheat kernel.

The dinner was prepared with lots of love and cooked with care so that everyone would eat at least a small portion of each of the foods served.

To prepare for the program, I used two large cookie sheets. One I filled with processed and refined foods. On the other I placed unprocessed highly nutritional foods as close as possible to the way nature made them. A tray on the left held sugar and refined, hydrogenated oils. In opposition, the tray on the right included foods that were pure and wholesome.

Here is the list of foods used:

First Cookie Sheet	*Second cookie sheet*
1. White bread	1. Wheat bread
2. White sugar	2. Honey
3. Brown sugar	3. Pure maple syrup
4. Candy bar	4. Seedless grapes
5. Canned soda	5. Orange
6. Potato chips	6. Sunflower seeds
7. Bubble gum	7. Wheat germ and bran
8. Peanut butter with hydrogenated oil and sugar	8. Natural peanut butter
9. Fruit pie	9. Garden tomato
10. Canned green beans	10. Garden green bean

This is the story as it actually happened on that Monday night in July. After the dishes were put in the dishwasher, the floor swept, and the table wiped clean, our children gathered in the family room.

After this lesson I expected that we would certainly have choices to make. I would set a good example by committing myself to buy and choose foods of more nutritional value. My family would make different food selections away from home.

The lesson began by having me tell each child how special they were to me. Each was told how they had many talents to help others. I explained that each one could accomplish great things in their lives and that they would be successful in reaching their goals.

Then I asked, "What does daddy put in the car to make it go?" "The key," 2-year-old David replied. "Yes, that is one thing he needs. But what does daddy pump into the car that is needed to make it move when daddy turns the key?" "Gas!" shouted Arlene. "That's right," I answered.

"What do you think would happen if daddy put water or soda in the car?" "It would choke to death," replied Bryan. "That is one way of putting it," I said. "The car surely would not run very well at first. Then the engine would stop. Gas and soda are both wet, but only gas has the right chemicals to keep the car running properly. Even if daddy uses the cheap gas, the spark plugs that help start the car have to be changed more often.

"This is just like our bodies. When we put a lot of junk food like candy, cookies, or empty-calorie foods in our bodies, they will finally run down and need lots of repairs. These repairs could include anything from tooth decay to tonsilitis. Cars go to the service station when they need repairs. People sometimes go to the hospital. If we want to keep our bodies healthy so we can accomplish our life goals, we would be very wise to be strong and turn down a lot of sugar-filled foods. We should eat them only occasionally."

I explained that I would no longer be buying empty-calorie foods. I brought back to their memory all the sickness we had the previous winter. They agreed to try changing our diet. We wanted to see if this would cut down the illness we had experienced.

The cookie sheets were introduced next. After talking about empty-calorie foods, the children immediately picked which cookie sheet had the good food and which had food that was not so good.

We played a game by mixing up items on the two trays. Then we had the children rearrange the items on the correct tray. We took the trays into another room. I challenged the children to remember what was on each tray, noting two categories of food—"Empty-Calorie Foods" and "Naturally Good Foods." They would tell me the item. Then they would tell me on which side to list it. This was a lot of fun, and since repetition usually teaches small children best we played the game twice.

The picture of the wheat kernel, which was taped to a small blackboard, was explained. The children were very surprised when I explained how bleached white flour was made. First, I held up the small packets of bran and said, "This is taken off," as I pointed to the skin on the wheat. "It is full of B vitamins which are for our nerves." Then I pointed to the germ and said, "This is taken out," while holding up a small bag of wheat germ. "The germ is full of vitamins E and B which are good for our blood and nerves." Then I pointed to the endosperm. I explained that after a lot of nature's vitamins were taken away from the wheat, and a bleaching agent added along with several man-made vitamins, the flour was then packaged to be sent to a store or to bakeries where white bread is made.

A feeling of success was in the room. The children were obviously touched and I was sure that they would soon be strengthened physically. For the next two weeks five little voices were heard repeating, "Is this good for you, mommy?" "Does this have sugar in it?" "Will this make me strong?" "Will I get sick if I eat this?" My idea worked! The children seemed to understand why I was not going to buy sugar-filled fruit pies, sweet chocolate cakes and squeezable, soft, white bread at the bakery anymore.

This is just one example of how to introduce your family to better nutrition. Older children might not be as receptive to the new change so the example you set and your patience can be the key to success as you apply the next 19 steps of better nutrition. You may find ways to bring good nutrition to your table without your older children even knowing what you have done.

There are many excellent books listed in the bibliography to help you. Just to put these steps into practice; to witness greater health and strength begin for your family will increase your convictions. As you continue with these steps, your heart will rejoice to know you and your family are eating properly so that they may have a better chance to live longer, healthier, and happier lives.

Chapter 4

Step 2
Whole-Wheat

Wheat is bread and bread is life. With bread, man goes on to build and explore. Without bread, famine steps in and great nations decline.

In times of prosperity, many people store food for use in hard times. There are those who will accuse such people of hoarding. But to store food in times of plenty is not hoarding. It is, rather, the stockpiling of foods which may become scarce. Wheat should be the backbone of any storage program because of the nutrition it supplies and because of its whole food value. Three hundred pounds of wheat per person has been recommended for a year's supply. If you do not store a year's supply of food at least store enough for small emergencies and every day use. Wheat should be used on a regular basis, not just when there is nothing else in the pantry or when grocery money is low.

Many people have developed unwise eating habits. Their taste buds are trained to accept only refined, devitalized foods. Circumstances which force them to eat more wheat from their food storage can be rewarding. To store wheat to eat only in hard times or famine while refined white flour continues to be eaten is a mistake. Let us see why.

First of all, your system takes time to adjust to whole-wheat. Diarrhea commonly occurs in those whose systems are not accustomed to a consumption of wheat flour in large quantities. Second, if you eat only refined flour you rob your body of many important B and E vitamins as well as others lost in the refining process. To learn of the many nutrients found in wheat is to understand why we hear it called "The Miracle of Wheat."

When broken down and analyzed, the wheat kernel is found to consist of three important parts:

1. The bran, or outer covering, makes up the skin of the wheat kernel. Bran is rich in precious B vitamins and minerals as well as in high-quality protein. Thousands of people have "bowel syndrome" which is a result of a lack of roughage in their diet. Bran can be the cure for this syndrome in nearly every case. Constipation can result when too many refined, carbohydrated foods form the main part of a diet. White bread, noodles, spaghetti, crackers and cookies lack bran that exists in the original whole-wheat. Bran can do far more to keep the doctor away than can the traditional apple a day. To return approximately two to three grams of crude fiber (about two to three heaping teaspoons of bran) to your diet can improve bowel behavior as well as prevent constipation. With bran a part of your diet you will become—and remain—regular.

2. The germ, or embryo, is where new life begins. Wheat-germ is one of the richest known sources of the B-complex vitamins and of vitamin E. Wheat-germ also contains protein, fat, and mineral matter. Both bran and the whole-wheat contain organic phosphates which provide brain and nerve food. Calcium for bones and teeth are also supplied from these parts of the wheat kernel.

Wheat-germ is an outstanding buy for all those who are searching to get the most nourishment for their money. It can be used in or on so many foods and dishes. Wheat-germ even makes creative cooking fun as you sprinkle it on cottage cheese, whipped cream, or cheese-topped casseroles.

Vitamin E, so richly found in wheat germ, is the "youth vitamin" . . . a vitamin which is completely destroyed in the processing of white, refined flour as well as in many of the refined oils. There are athletes who attribute their skill and stamina to the use of wheat-germ or vitamin E. There are those who have suffered heart attacks and who now take vitamin E on the advice of their doctor.[2] It puts oxygen in the blood and is known as the "healing vitamin." To take the germ from wheat may take youth, health, and physical endurance from the consumer.

3. The endosperm makes up the larger portion of the wheat kernel. Cellulose, starch, gluten are most abundant in the endosperm. Vitamin or mineral substance is present in small quantities. Protein is the main ingredient in the endosperm from which white flour is primarily made.

Fat from the wheat kernel has a high food value since it also contains unsaturated fatty acids. It is important to eat the complete kernel in order to receive the full value from wheat.

---

2. Wilfrid E. Shute, *Vitamin E for Ailing and Healthy Hearts*.

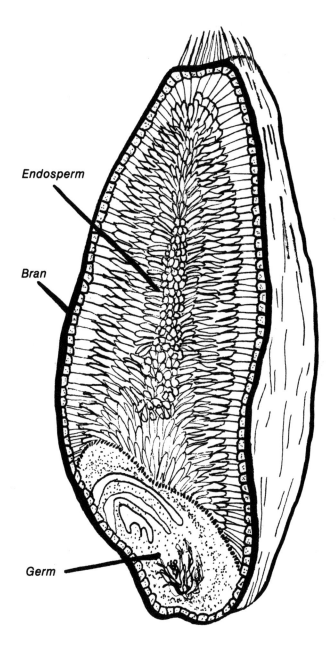

Endosperm

Bran

Germ

A Wheat Kernel
"The Miracle Made for Man"
Drawing by Kandace Cleland

Now that you know why whole-wheat is such a treasure, you should also understand why wheat can be more valuable than gold, especially in times of famine. You cannot eat gold. Wheat should be part of your daily diet and part of your food storage as well.

Many families put away a year's supply of wheat. Knowing that wheat can be stored for long periods of time, these families save the wheat for a rainy day. To store wheat and not use it is like waiting to enjoy your fortune after you die. Even though wheat can be stored for long periods, the importance of eating what you store cannot be overemphasized. Stored whole-wheat should be rotated with fresh wheat on a regular basis.

The following true story will emphasize the importance of using your wheat on a day-to-day basis.

Store What You Eat and Eat What You Store

A military family we will call Brian and Sherri Stone purchased one thousand pounds of red winter wheat. The wheat had been specially treated, then placed in heavy, plastic bags and sealed in round metal cans. The wheat was put away by the Stones in case of emergency as part of their food storage plan.

The Stones were not especially fond of whole-wheat because they had not acquired a taste for it. In fact, Sherri Stone had never made a recipe using whole-wheat flour, but to store wheat seemed the right thing to do.

The Stone family did realize that if you do not eat, you do not live. Sherri decided that if the need should arise she would use her one wheat recipe book to hurriedly teach herself how to adapt to wheat cookery.

At first the cans of wheat sat in their home. With bright colored covers they were used as end tables. But after three years they were put in a garage where the cans were exposed to temperature changes.

Brian and Sherri Stone did not worry about the wheat since they checked it once a year for unwanted weevil. The wheat appeared to be as beautiful as it was the day they bought it. As they checked their valuable possession, the Stones felt as if they would never go hungry.

Since the Stone family moved six times because of military orders, their wheat cost them an extra $600 for being overweight on their household goods. The Stone family was trying to do what they thought was right, but they did not follow the plan to store what you eat and eat what you store.

Then disaster struck in the form of unexpected bills. The savings of the Stone family were wiped out, extras were cut completely and the grocery money suffered severely. The Stones decided their stored wheat would truly be a help to get them through this financial squeeze.

For breakfast Sherri included cracked-wheat cereal on the menu. Long faces appeared as each child tasted the cereal. Evidently a chemical change had taken place during the storing of the wheat because of the kind of plastic bag used and the wheat had taken on the taste of the bag. Brian Stone ended up by selling the wheat at ten cents a pound to a farmer for chicken feed.

The Stone family found from others who had stored their wheat for long periods that they, too, had their mishaps. Many had lost their wheat to the little brown weevil bug. Others lost their wheat to mold. Sherri Stone decided to learn how to use wheat in her cooking on a regular basis so she would be prepared to use it should another emergency occur.

Wheat is so important in your diet that you need not only plan to store it but to learn how to make it a part of your everyday diet. Use wheat daily. You will benefit in the following ways:

1. *Physically*—Your body will be receiving much needed B and E vitamins.

2. *Emotionally*—Having already developed the skills in using wheat will be a blessing.

3. *Temporally*—You can know how much wheat your family needs for a year if you actually use it.

You may think of using your wheat to make bread or cracked-wheat cereal. To make whole-wheat bread can be a challenge and it takes practice, since both texture and process are different than white bread. Homemakers should be strongly encouraged to make their own bread. This is one of the best ways to use your wheat storage. To read ingredients labels and prices for commercial whole-wheat bread should be enough to convince you that homemade bread contains better ingredients and is less expensive as well. To make your own bread takes only a little effort and the rewards are great.

If your family is not accustomed to whole-wheat, try the transitional bread recipe (p. 118) which uses unbleached white flour. Gradually add more whole-wheat flour each time you make bread. Try adding a small amount of soy flour to your recipe. This will give extra nutrition and keep the bread moist as well.

The overnight method of bread baking (p. 119) will be a great help to busy mothers who find it hard to schedule time for bread making; or make enough bread to last for a week. Put the family to work on this project. Making bread can be both fun and satisfying.

If there are reasons why you cannot make your own bread, purchase *whole*-wheat bread but be aware that bread labeled "wheat bread" is not *whole*-wheat bread. Again, read labels: you will see the difference.

You can also serve cracked-wheat cereal and make whole-wheat pancakes. Use some whole-wheat flour when baking recipes that call for flour. Once you and your family acquire a taste for whole-wheat flour, you may find that white flour tastes bland.

To grind flour on your baking day will help make you ready for the next week's baking. Start by grinding five pounds of whole-wheat flour and at least a quart of cracked-wheat cereal. These can be kept in your refrigerator or freezer.

Chapter 5

Step 3
Cereals

"Please pass the Sugar Snaps." "Did you buy any Sugar Crunch?" "Where are the Coco-Crackles?" "Who ate all the Fruit-flavored Corn Balls?" Are these the first cereals chosen at your breakfast table?

After your study of nutrition and the story of wheat created for man, you can begin to make transitional changes. Breakfast is a good place to start because that meal begins to provide the fuel which gives your body the needed energy for the day.

Many mothers, sadly uninformed about the importance of giving their bodies proper fuel to begin the day, will skip breakfast themselves. Their children receive a convenient bowl of packaged cereal but some boxed cereals can actually be listed as "empty-calorie" foods.

Sugar is listed as the second ingredient in many cereals after stripped wheat, toasted corn, or popped rice. Still, there are mothers who start the morning on a sweet note as they serve roasted and toasted sugar cereals, pastry pop-ups which are filled with preserves and one-minute oatmeal sweetened with empty-calorie refined sugar.

These grains are stripped of their skin and germ which contain most of the nutritive value.[3] Natural vitamins created in the grains are left on the floor of the refiner's factory or sold in your health food store in bags with the labels of wheat germ and bran. Refining robs the breakfast cereals of vitamin E and the B-complex vitamins. It also takes away some protein and unsaturated fatty acids. After the refiners have processed the grain and taken out nature-made vitamins and minerals, the grain is enriched, or fortified, with synthetic vitamins. The cereal producers "fortify" because refining has destroyed almost everything.

---

3. Gary Null, *The New Vegetarian*, p. 169.

Eight or ten synthetic vitamins, sometimes minerals, are put back into cereal. Although vitamins are restored, enzymes are not. You be the judge. Are the breakfast cereals you give your family enriched or are they robbed? Why settle for eight or ten essential vitamins when you can have all the vitamins and minerals that were intended for your body by serving cracked-wheat cereal, whole-wheat pancakes, and whole-wheat toast for breakfast?

Start the transition process by purchasing only cereals with less than 10 percent sugar. Raisin Bran is a good cereal to buy while you are switching over to whole grains. Even though it has nine grams of sugar, four of these are found, naturally, in the raisins. Cheerios, Grape Nuts, and Wheat Chex are also good cereals for transition. When using cold cereals, one to two teaspoons of bran and one to two teaspoons wheat germ may be added for extra nutrition. You may hide this easily in Raisin Bran. If you need additional sweetener, try a bit of pure maple syrup or honey.

Among cereals which contain 10 percent sugar or less are: Cheerios, 2.7 percent; Puffed Rice, 2.8 percent; Wheat Chex, 3.5 percent; Grape Nut Flakes, 3.9 percent; Post Toasties, 5.8 percent; Product 19, 5.8 percent; Corn Total, 5.8 percent; Wheaties, 8.9 percent; Corn Flakes, 9.1 percent; and Crispy Rice, 8.8 percent. Compare these to Fruit Pebbles, 56.2 percent, King Vitamin 61.6 percent, and Sugar Smacks, 63.7 percent sugar.[4] (There are even some cereals with no sugar added which include Shredded Wheat and Grape Nuts.)

It is very important to check each label before you spend your food dollars. Consider purchasing only items which place sugar no higher than fourth on the ingredients list. After you have changed all cereals to those with less than 10 percent sugar, your family may develop a taste for cracked-wheat cereal which has many of the B vitamins. It is also very chewy and very filling. Both whole-wheat and cracked-wheat cereals cook wonderfully in a crockpot. Getting enough B vitamins will calm your nerves while helping you get rid of your sweet tooth that sneakily puts on those extra pounds.

A bit of honey, blackstrap molasses, or pure maple syrup and butter all taste delicious with cracked-wheat cereal (p. 118). After the wheat is cracked, store it in the refrigerator or freezer to keep its freshness and also to keep out bugs.

Homemade granola (p. 118) is a delicious treat for breakfast. Making a big batch is a breeze. It can be made in bulk and stored in

---

4. Ira L. Shannon, D.M.D., M.S.D., "Should They Be Called Imitation Cereals?" *The Journal of Denistry for Children*, Sept. - Oct. 1974.

a large plastic container in the refrigerator. Consider serving granola one day of each week. Then surprise your family with the lightest whole-wheat pancakes (p. 119) ever. Why not make Saturday pancake day at your house? It could be the incentive to help children get up and do their chores quickly.

After mastering this step, you will hear sweet voices in the morning saying, "Please pass the granola." "Did you make enough cracked-wheat cereal for two bowls?" "Where is the pure maple syrup?" "Who ate all the whole-wheat pancakes? I only got one!"

Chapter 6

Step 4
Junk Food

Sally Jones had just delivered her third baby in three years. She noticed that twenty-three extra pounds had sneaked onto her young figure. She blamed it on her pregnancies and lack of exercise but she had second thoughts when she saw a picture of a round, plump lady. The lady had before her an ice cream sundae. Sally realized she ate her own share of sweets.

Sally Jones cut out the picture of the overweight lady. She taped it on her refrigerator door to remind her that you are what you eat. Sally knew she was no exception, that she had no right to judge. Her diet began immediately. She lost twenty pounds by dieting, by exercising, and by looking daily at the truth-revealing picture hanging on her refrigerator door. The picture kept her motivated until she reached her goal.

Let's see how, through proper nutrition, Sally's overweight could have been prevented in the first place.

Junk food can be classified into three categories: (1) dead, (2) refined, or (3) preserved with additives. Junk food adds weight to your body almost faster than the revealed truth shows on your scales. To eat more fiber such as that in raw vegetables can satisfy hunger pains and help stifle the temptation to eat junk foods. This one idea would have helped Sally Jones keep her weight down.

Reading labels is a magic formula to help you accomplish your goal in this "Junk Foods" step. Watch for refined sugar, refined white flour, hydrogenated oils, preservatives and artificial color and flavorings. We are fooled and robbed every day as we spend food dollars on empty calorie junk foods.

Here is a list of common junk food to be found in a supermarket. Count. See how many of these items will be fooling your body as well as robbing your grocery dollars.

List of Junk Foods

1. Brownie mixes
2. Brown sugar
3. Cakes (packaged, frozen or bakery)
4. Candy (made with chocolate or refined sugar)
5. Canned fruit with heavy syrup
6. Cereals (prepackaged, instant and sweetened)
7. Chocolate chips
8. Chocolate powder or syrup
9. Cookies (store bought)
10. Crackers
11. Flavored gelatin
12. Frosting mixes (boxed or canned)
13. Frozen dinners
14. Frozen waffles, pancakes, french toast, etc.
15. Fruit juices (those which are sugared)
16. Hydrogenated oils
17. Ice cream
18. Imitation maple syrup
19. Jams and jellies
20. Marshmallows
21. Pastries
22. Peanuts (roasted in containers with preservatives)
23. Pies
24. Potato chips
25. Pretzels
26. Puddings (boxed or canned)
27. Soda pop
28. Squeeze cheese
29. Toaster pastries
30. White bread (bleached white flour)
31. White sugar

Use these items in moderation. This will be a start. Moderation can fit perfectly the times you and your family get these unremembered goodies at church socials, birthday parties, friends' homes and in many school lunches. This happens almost every day so it will be better to remove the temptation of empty-calorie foods from the home.

Surprisingly, many people feel that these foods are nutritionally good for them. They believe they can't buy anything in a store which will harm their bodies. This is not always true.

When one over-indulges in junk foods, patience is shortened. Did you ever think to blame overweight on the inability to control unruly tastebuds? Many of the excess pounds overweight people have might have been prevented had good eating habits been established when they were children. Many uninformed mothers actually train their children to rely on sweets by using them as a pacifier: "If you don't cry," or "If you pick up your toys I will give you a cookie." Habits like these, along with the many empty-calorie foods from which to choose, have contributed to the weight problem which approximately one-third of all American people have.

To reward ourselves with sugar-filled goodies satisfies only for the moment. We can regret our actions later when depression sets in.

Eating out excessively can also be harmful to our bodies since much restaurant food falls into the junk-food category. A mother may say, "I will buy a milkshake instead of soda for my child. It's better for him." How amazing! The truth is that milkshakes at too many hamburger stands are made of one-third hydrogenated oil, plenty of sugar, artificial flavoring and milk powder mixed with water. And these same franchise drive-in hamburgers contain one tablespoon of sugar per hamburger, including what is in the bread and catsup. Still, more people eat out now than ever before. It would be terrific if there were more restaurants serving fresh fruits and vegetables. Moderation in all things is a good general rule which should apply to eating out, too. As a real treat, eating out has its proper place.

A list of alternative choices to junk food is included to help you with your grocery list. In addition, almost anything you can grow in a garden can replace nearly all of the junk foods.

Alternatives to Junk Food

1. Apples
2. Bananas
3. Bell peppers
4. Carob powder (to make brownies and candy)
5. Carob chips (to replace chocolate chips)
6. Celery sticks
7. Dates or any dried fruit
8. Cherries
9. Grapes
10. Fruit-nut mix
11. Grape juice (without sugar)
12. Graham cracker (made with honey, found at health food stores)

13. Honey Candy
14. Nuts
15. Oranges
16. Orange Julius (peach, pineapple, or strawberry, too!)
17. Peanuts in the shell
18. Peanut butter (natural)
19. Plums in season
20. Popcorn (try with powdered cheddar cheese)
21. Prunes
22. Raisins
23. Sunflower seeds
24. Tomatoes
25. White cheese sticks
26. Yogurt

Now that you know what to feed your family, eliminate as many junk foods as possible from your grocery list. Knowing what to feed your family is good but getting them to partake is the real challenge. Encourage in your family strong, positive desires to live long lives in good health. Eliminate or cut down all junk foods. Use a positive approach to retrain their taste buds so that they will shy away from salty and sugar-filled foods. Decide it is time to take charge of what you and your family eat.

Usually, the mother buys the family's groceries. If cookies, brownies, soda and ice cream are not purchased, cookies, brownies, soda and ice cream will not be eaten. When the children ask for snacks or treats, they can choose between fruit, nuts or a nutritious homemade snack. You won't have to worry about whether your family is eating junk food at home because there won't be any there for them to eat.

Consider making treats this week from the recipe section to serve your family. You don't need to remark on how nutritious the treats are. For you to know you are giving your family needed vitamins should be enough.

Here is a list of items to be used by a mother who cares. This list includes what she will use to make health-giving changes in her every-day cooking.

The Mother Who Cares Includes In Her Food Storage:
1. Raw honey
2. Date sugar
3. Blackstrap molasses
4. Pure maple syrup
5. Whole-wheat flour (stone-ground)

6. Unbleached white flour
7. Carob powder
8. Brown rice
9. Wheat germ
10. Soy flour
11. Brewer's yeast
12. Sesame seeds (unhulled)
13. Sunflower seeds (raw)
14. Kelp (used as a salt substitute)
15. Iodized sea salt
16. Unsweetened coconut
17. Seeds for sprouting
18. Raw nuts

Many of these foods can be bought at health food stores. It is not called a "health food store" to scare you away. Most food sold there helps to keep the body healthy. However, even health food stores may have junk foods on their shelves—read labels.

The Mother Who Cares Eliminates From Her Food Storage:

1. Bleached white flour
2. Refined sugar
3. Canned soda pop
4. All sugar cereals
5. Flavored gelatin, pudding, cake and brownie mixes
6. White rice
7. Fruits canned in heavy syrup
8. Hydrogenated peanut butter
9. All candy made with refined sugar
10. Refined table salt
11. Any product containing BHA or BHT (preservatives which have been banned in England)
12. Hydrogenated shortenings (solid at room temperature)
13. Maraschino cherries (contain many preservatives)
14. All synthetic sweeteners and products sweetened with them (such as cyclamates and saccharin)
15. Commercial breads that are loaded with emulsifiers and preservatives

Eliminating junk food is one of the most important steps outlined in this book because it might be the hardest eating habit to change. Habit is a powerful influence. In most cases, your habits may have to be changed so drastically that it might take a year or more to completely adjust to the new way you spend your grocery dollars.

Each junk food you eliminate from your grocery list will bring you that much closer to a successful change. As you master this step, place a circle around each item on the junk-food list which you have successfully cut from your grocery buying.

As you witness the decrease of colds, flu, headaches, and other minor sicknesses in your home, convictions will turn to knowledge. You will find it easier to stay away from junk food and empty-calorie food outside the home. The children may still have their sugar-filled treats at school or church, but remember: you have the stewardship in the home. Your example which extends outside the home will also be important. When your daughter follows your example by saying to her friend "No, thank you" when offered a piece of candy or when your son thanks you during the year for preparing food that helps him have a strong body, how great shall be your reward!

Chapter 7

Step 5
Honey

Waking to the sound of her radio, a young mother heard an announcer say, "... most nutritionists agree—sugar consumption in America needs to be reduced. The average American consumes a hundred and fifty pounds of sugar a year."

A quick mathematical check will show that each person, on the average, consumes seven-eighths cup of sugar every day for one year. If that is not enough to make you question your sugar intake, to think what sugar may be doing to your body should.

The refining of sugar cane into white sugar strips the sugar of nutrients and makes it an empty-calorie food.

Sugar has many adverse effects on your body. Assimilation of vitamins is affected; elimination of bacteria from your body is hampered; chance of heart attack and other ailments may be increased and blood-sugar level is lowered by the consumption of too much sugar!

Since sugar is stripped of vitamins, minerals and essential amino acids it lacks the very B vitamins and minerals necessary for its assimilation so that your body must take vitamins from other foods or storage depots in your body to serve this purpose which could result in a B-complex vitamin and mineral deficiency.[5] So we see that the sugar you eat actually takes away value from wholesome foods by requiring your body to use its own assimilated nutrients to metabolize the sugar.[6] Also, calcium may not be absorbed well when too much sugar is eaten.[7]

---

5. "Sugar: The Facts Are More Sour Than Sweet." *Nutrition Now!* March 1980, p. 1, 3.
6. *Ibid.*
7. *Ibid.*

If you eat too much sugar you may well reduce your intake of fiber and fiber aids in the process of carrying bacteria to the intestines.[8] These bacteria are then eliminated in your stool. The more sugar you eat, the less bacteria will be in the stool. Bacteria thus left in your bowel has the potential to damage your body. Chances of a heart attack may be greatly increased by the intake of large amounts of sugar.[9] Arthritis, hypertension, diabetes, obesity and tooth decay are among the diseases being linked to eating too much sugar.

Even if you do not want to cut sugar from your diet completely, the amount you consume can be drastically reduced. And sugar can also contribute to low blood-sugar which in medical terms is known as "hypoglycemia."[10] Symptoms of hypoglycemia are migraine headaches, hyperactivity, obesity, fatigue, trembling, anxiety, depression, allergies, cold sweats, dizziness, fainting spells, forgetfulness, drowsiness and arthritic pains.

Hypoglycemia causes late-morning and afternoon cravings for snacks. Drowsiness, mild depression, and a trembling feeling may result. "Hunger pains" may indicate a low blood-sugar level instead of an empty stomach.

Hypoglycemics should avoid refined sugars, caffeine, nicotine and alcohol.[11] A high-protein diet helps break the cycle. The craving for sugar ceases and the blood can maintain a normal glucose level.[12]

One mother exclaimed, "I never knew eating too much sugar could hurt your body. I always thought it did not matter so long as you ate plenty of good food, too." If you begin to see a need to eat less sugar perhaps you are wondering how to cut down. To eliminate sugar completely can cause withdrawal symptoms because the use of sugar can be addictive, so this method is not recommended. To cut back gradually on the amount eaten is preferable.

Many mothers claim they hardly use white sugar at all. They insist that they bought five pounds of sugar ages ago and still have half of the bag left. Yet they fail to realize how sneaky food processors have been. Commercially processed and refined food are often more than 50 percent sugar. The U.S. Department of Agriculture says that to avoid sugar consumption is difficult. In 1920, 60 percent of the sugar Americans ate was added to the food by the consumer. Today, 75 percent of the sugar we eat is added by food processors.

8. *Ibid.*
9. Gary Null, *The New Vegetarian*, p. 274.
10. *Ibid.*, p. 272.
11. *Ibid.*, p. 272, 273.
12. *Ibid.*

Learn to read labels at the grocery store. If sugar is listed before the third or fourth ingredient, that item should be replaced with a better brand. Homemade items are better yet. Remember that corn syrup, corn syrup solids, dextrose, sucrose, maltose and lactose are all used as other names for sugar.

In most convenience foods, sugar is a major ingredient. Peanut butter, pickles, spaghetti sauce, frozen dinners, frozen pizzas, salad dressings, gelatin desserts, canned fruits and vegetables, hot dogs and imitation powder drinks all contain sugar which help add up to the seven-eighths cup of sugar per day we are said to consume. These items can easily be replaced with your homemade products. (This will be discussed in the "Getting Organized" section of this book.)

Honey may replace sugar in much of your baking. Although honey should not be eaten to excess either, since too much honey can cause obesity and tooth decay, it is still far superior to sugar.

"My son eat thou honey because it is good; and the honeycomb, which is sweet to thy taste" (Proverbs 24:13). Honey contains fructose which is the natural sweetner also found in fruits and glucose. Honey requires no conversion since it can be absorbed directly into the bloodstream through the stomach wall.

The honey you use should be unheated and unfiltered to ensure that all natural enzymes and vitamins are still present. Honey found in supermarkets has been heated to provide longer shelf life.

Honey can replace sugar in most recipes. When a recipe calls for one cup sugar, three-fourths cup honey can be used instead; next time one-half cup honey; then one-fourth cup honey. As your tastes change, even a little honey may seem very sweet.

As you try to get away from sugar to the use of more natural sweetness, remember how our culture is centered around sugar. To cut back on your sugar intake may not be easy unless you make an alternative plan.

Think of the holidays—almost one a month—which center around sugary treats: New Year's Day, Valentine's, Easter, Mother's Day, Father's Day, Fourth of July, Labor Day, Halloween, Thanksgiving and Christmas, as well as individual birthdays. To start new, more nutritious traditions for these holidays will take imagination and creativity. Some good ideas could include heart-shaped boxes for Valentine's Day filled with homemade goodies (p. 134). Easter baskets could be filled with the traditional colored eggs and honey candy (p. 132). Fourth of July can be celebrated with a traditional cook-out. Instead of hot dogs and potato chips, try grilled fish with skewered vegetables. For dessert serve homemade ice cream (p. 133).

For Halloween have an old-fashioned party at home. Bobbing for apples is always fun. Refreshments of honey popcorn balls (p. 133) and apple cider could be served.

Thanksgiving is usually a nutritious meal with turkey, dressing made with whole-wheat bread and whole-wheat corn brean (p. 117), sweet potatoes candied with pure maple syrup, and fruit salad (p. 128). The traditional desserts would have to be changed very little to make them more nutritious. The pumpkin and pecan pies (p. 134, 135) are delightful for dessert.

Christmas can still be fun even when fewer treats are served. Start to collect recipes with good wholesome ingredients or make changes in those you already have. Try stuffing stockings with large juicy oranges and peanuts still in the shell.

As you think through these holidays, you will come up with many ideas of your own. Consider cutting back nightly desserts to once-a-week treats. Have fun, and remember . . . eating less sugar won't be as boring as you might think.

Chapter 8

Step 6
Protein

Those days when your protein intake is inadequate are the days when your body grows older. Protein is an important part of your diet. Only water is more plentiful in your body than protein. Protein is made of eight essential amino acids. These amino acids repair worn-out tissue and help to build new tissue. An adequate supply is needed daily.

Protein may be obtained from many sources: beef, poultry, fish, dried beans, eggs, milk, cheese, buttermilk, yogurt, brewer's yeast and peanut butter all contain protein. All parts of your body are maintained by the protein which you consume.

Breakfast is a very important meal since protein provides your body fuel for the day. The less protein eaten in the morning the sooner a mid-morning lag comes on. Tests have proven that those who consume at least twenty-two grams of protein for breakfast have energy to last through the day.

How do you plan a breakfast which will contain twenty-two grams of protein? Knowing how many grams of protein there are in each food will help.[13]

Source	Amount	Grams of Protein
Beans		
Great Northern	½ cup, cooked	6.6
Green Pea Soup	½ cup	4.3
Kidney	½ cup, cooked	7.2
Lima	½ cup, cooked	6.5
Lentils	½ cup, cooked	7.9
Mung	½ cup, raw	25.4
Navy	½ cup, cooked	7.5
Pinto	½ cup, cooked	6.6
Soybeans	½ cup, cooked	30.0

13. Barbara Kraus, *The Barbara Kraus Dictionary of Protein.*

Source	Amount	Grams of Protein
Beef		
Chuck Roast	4 ounces	29.5
Ground		
Regular	4 ounces	27.4
Lean	4 ounces	31.1
Liver	4 ounces	29.9
Rump Roast	4 ounces	26.8
Steak		
Club	4 ounces	23.4
Sirloin	4 ounces	25.2
T-bone	4 ounces	22.1
Bread		
White	1 ounce slice	2.5
Whole-wheat	1 ounce slice	2.9
Brewer's Yeast	1 tablespoon	3.1
Cereals		
Millet (uncooked)	1 cup	11.2
Oatmeal	1 cup	11.5
Soy Grits	1 cup	56.9
Cheese		
Cheddar	1 ounce	7.1
Colby	1 ounce	7.0
Cottage	1 ounce	3.75
Cream	1 ounce	2.3
Mozarella	1 ounce	8.0
Parmesan	1 ounce	10.2
Chicken (cooked)	4 ounces	27.0
Egg (boiled)	1 large	6.4
Fish		
Cod	4 ounces	32.2
Haddock	4 ounces	26.3
Perch	4 ounces	23.3
Salmon	4 ounces	18.5
Shrimp	4 ounces	17.4
Tuna (canned in water)	4 ounces	31.6

Source	Amount	Grams of Protein
Flour		
Carob	1 ounce	1.3
Corn	1 ounce	2.2
Rye	1 ounce	3.0
Soybean	1 ounce	13.2
Whole-wheat	1 ounce	3.8
White	1 ounce	3.0
Milk		
Whole	1 cup	8.4
Skim	1 cup	10.3
Instant	1 cup	8.0
Non-instant	1 cup	16.0
Buttermilk	1 cup	8.8
Nuts		
Almonds (chopped)	1 cup	23.6
Peanuts (raw)	1 cup	60.0
Pecans (chopped)	1 cup	9.6
Walnuts (chopped)	1 cup	33.6
Peanut Butter	1 tablespoon	4.4
Rice		
Brown	½ cup	2.8
Sunflower Seeds	½ cup	14.7
Tofu	4.2 ounces	9.4
Turkey	4 ounces	37.3
Wheat Germ	½ cup	30.0
Yogurt	½ cup	4.1

Total up grams of protein for each day to at least sixty grams for women, seventy grams for men, and forty to one hundred grams for growing children depending on their age. More grams are needed after they reach the age of twelve because of rapid growth. At least twenty-two of these protein grams should be eaten for breakfast. This will give a good start for a happier day and a healthier body.

Beef

Beef contains about 22 percent protein as well as iron and several B vitamins. While you do get nutrition from meat, let us examine what cattle raisers are doing to their cattle: eighty percent are being fattened by DES. This is a femal hormone which increases the weight of cattle, but it produces fat rather than protein.

Antibiotics are used to fight animal diseases and they also make cattle grow faster. Antibiotic residues are not destroyed by cooking. As a result the meat you eat may make you more susceptible to certain infections.

You may want to find a cattle-raiser who does not use DES or antibiotics. Most American families could easily cut back on the amount of beef consumed. Other sources of protein may be substituted.

Organ meats from beef are its best nutritional sources. One wise mother uses a mixture of two pounds ground beef, one pound heart, and one pound lung all ground together. This gives her four pounds of nutritious meat for less than what she would pay for ground beef. She uses it in any dish as she would regular ground beef.

Another mother uses only half the ground beef called for in a recipe. She then serves cheese or eggs with the meal to ensure adequate protein.

Beef liver (p. 124) is a good source of iron as well as vitamin A. Many people will not eat liver because they find the taste objectionable. If your family is young, tell them you are having a special kind of meat that makes you strong. They will enjoy the meal and never be any the wiser.

Beef does supply necessary protein, but careful consideration will need to be given to decide how much beef is to be included in your diet. You may be pleasantly surprised to find there are other sources of complete protein which cost considerably less than beef.

For instance, one tortilla shell and three-fourths cup pinto beans contain eleven grams of protein and all eight essential amino acids. Cream of potato soup can be a complete protein and so can peanut butter served on whole-wheat bread. As all eight essential amino acids are needed, it does not matter from where they come. It does not matter which amino acid comes from what food. You only need to be concerned that you get the right amount.

As you learn how to provide adequate protein, you will find it easier to eat less and less meat—an eating habit that may well add years to your life.

Poultry

Turkey is traditional for a Thanksgiving or Christmas dinner. It can also be enjoyed at other times of the year because it is such a good source of protein. Turkey is 56 percent protein compared to 22 percent protein in beef. Turkey has the lowest fat content of all meats and is relatively low in calories.

Other poultry can also supply quality protein: ducks are 38 percent protein, geese 41 percent and chickens are 20 percent protein.

The skin of poultry should be avoided, since it contains much of the fat. Broth from poultry may be saved for soup-making, but should be skimmed for fat after refrigeration.

Poultry is better for you than beef, but still does not need to be consumed in large quantities. You can make the most of the protein in poultry by serving it once a week. Many interesting ways can be devised to make your poultry dishes appealing.

Fish

In selecting meat protein, fish, poultry and then beef should be served. Fish contains more usable protein than does meat.

Fish has been used for centuries as an important protein source. After Jesus' resurrection, as he met with the apostles, he partook of fish and honeycomb. Even two thousand years before Christ, stalls were set up on the streets to sell fish to passersby. Today fish is often expensive, but it can be well worth the price because of its nutritional value.

Fresh fish is the best buy and is to be found in many grocery stores. Use care in purchasing frozen breaded fish. This fish often contains up to 50 percent bread. Canned fish such as tuna, salmon or sardines are a good buy because they are often of higher quality than frozen fish. Learn different ways to prepare fish and serve it more often to benefit your family.

Pork

Although pork contains protein, iron and small amounts of B vitamins, you may want to consider avoiding it. Pork is not only hard to digest (it can remain up to nine hours in the stomach), but it has a high amount of salt.[14] Salt is used by the food processors to kill trichinella spiralis worms which cause trichinosis. Consumption of pork which has been processed with salt has even been linked to migraine headaches and high blood pressure in some people.

---

14. J. I. Rodale, *The Complete Book of Food and Nutrition*, p.249.

Bacon is a staple food in many American homes. Besides having very little nutrition, bacon today is preserved with nitrates. Nitrates are being proven to cause health problems and even, in extreme cases, death.[15] Much thought will need to be given as to how bacon can be replaced as a traditional morning entree.

In the good old days, to eat hot dogs on a picnic was probably all right. Today when you have a hot dog, you are paying for a product which contains little protein. Most hot dogs contain pork, but even those made from beef are full of additives.

Research show that the average hot dog contains 60 percent moisture, 30 to 40 percent fat and 7 percent protein. In addition, your hot dog may contain artificial flavor, monosodium glutamate and nitrates as preservatives along with sugar, dextrose, water and a wide variety of "animal products" such as beef lip, pork lip, snout, tail-gristle, blood, lung, spleen, tripe and stomach.

Consider replacing your hot dog night with a more nutritious meal which will better benefit your family. Some health food stores sell hot dogs made from pure beef, but be prepared to pay extra for these—beef costs more than fillers.

As you make your grocery list, you would do well to eliminate lunch meats, hot dogs, bacon, ham, sausage and pork chops. Most lunch meats contain pork. Even if they don't, they are still full of additives and preservatives which do nothing to ensure your health.

Beans

There are many varieties of beans from which to choose. Black beans, black-eyed peas, chick-peas, navy beans, kidney beans, lentils, mung beans, pinto beans, split peas and soy beans may be used in a variety of ways.

Beans, or legumes, are an inexpensive source of protein, minerals and vitamins. Stretch your food dollar by serving beans more often.

Certain varieties of beans are bypassed because of the "gas" which can result from eating beans such as the "Pinto." Avoid this unpleasant reaction by sprouting the beans for two days prior to cooking. (Tips on sprouting found in Chapter 20.) Not only will the nutritional value be increased, but "gas" will no longer be a problem.

Even when beans don't need to be sprouted they will probably need to be soaked overnight before cooking which makes the beans more tender and shortens cooking time. If you forget to soak the beans, add one cup of beans to four cups of water and bring to a boil

---

15. Gary Null, The New Vegetarian, p. 83.

for one minute. Remove the pot from the stove and cover. Leave the beans for about one hour then simmer until done. Salt should be added after the beans are soft because salt takes out the moisture. Include beans often in your menu planning, not only to help your budget but to give your family their nutritional values.

A good protein breakfast will help your diet program. Since protein stays with you longer you won't get hungry again so soon.

Avoid mid-morning crankiness and irritability by starting your day with a high protein breakfast.

Do you find yourself reminding your child to stand up straight? Have you noticed your own posture lately? If stooped shoulders are a problem with anyone in your family, not eating enough protein could be a factor.

Great care should be used in planning your menus to ensure that adequate protein is included. An egg for breakfast and meat for dinner will not provide your body with the protein it needs. The protein chart gives the content of different foods to help you plan your menus. Always keep in mind the fact that protein is too important a nutrient to be neglected.

Chapter 9

Step 7
Peanut Butter and Salt

Peanut Butter

This step will be one of the easiest to master. When you buy your next jar of peanut butter, simply make sure it contains 100 percent peanuts. Many national brands contain only pure peanuts. Some supermarkets even make their own natural peanut butter and health food stores carry a good supply. Read your labels to know whether you are buying pure peanut butter or peanut butter mixed with hydrogenated oil and sugar.

Natural peanut butter will have natural peanut oil floating on top. Stir this oil in thoroughly, use the amount desired, then refrigerate to help keep the oils from separating and going rancid.

Many commercial brands of peanut butter contain as much as two-thirds hydrogenated oil (shortening) which is what makes them spread so smoothly. Commercial brands may also contain stabilizers, preservatives and as much as 10 percent sugar. These extra ingredients are neither necessary nor desirable.

How much nutrition do you think you get when you serve a peanut butter sandwich on white bread with jelly along with an imitation fruit drink? You get about twelve grams of protein and a lot of sugar. Now put natural peanut butter and honey on whole-wheat bread, add a glass of milk (non-instant powdered) and you will get twenty-seven grams of complete protein and a nutritious lunch.

A fun treat to give your children after school could be a peanut butter lollipop. Simply fill a teaspoon full of peanut butter and introduce the "peanut butter pop." Try No-Bake Peanut Butter Cookies (p. 133). If you get the whole family involved in rolling the cookies into balls and rolling them in the coconut, it could become a favorite family treat.

Let your little ones be creative with Peanut Butter Clay (p. 134). They will be using self-expression as they play and they will have a nutritious snack at the same time. Put a piece of waxed paper under the clay to keep the oil from getting on the table. A rolling pin and cookie cutters can be used in the play. With a little help from you, your children will receive a good source of protein along with a fun time.

Salt

Salt is added for taste to almost every commercially prepared food. Because salt is inorganic in nature, it cannot be assimilated by your body. Avoid purchasing foods with added salt by reading food labels. Already you have cut back on a considerable amount of salt consumption if you stopped eating salty junk foods as listed in Step 4.

A lot of high blood pressure is the result of too much salt in the diet. Many pregnant women are advised by their doctor to cut out salt and drink more liquids. Salt causes your body to retain water. It can poison the mother when toxemia develops.

Iodine is usually added to salt, but iodine can be found naturally in nature's foods. You merely need to eat more fish which contains iodine; use less salt.

If you feel you need extra flavoring when cooking, kelp, iodized sea salt or herb seasoning could be used like great grandma did. These will provide flavor without adding salt. Kelp and herb seasonings contain trace minerals. Kelp even has iodine.

A good rule to follow is if salt is used when cooking, it should not be used on the table. If you prefer to use salt on the table, don't use it while cooking. Veg-Salt may be purchased at a health food store which contains half sea salt and half vegetable seasonings.

To start the transition, you may become aware of all the salt you actually eat in one day. Then when you go to a health food store try organic, iodized sea salt and kelp.

Only if the weather is extremely hot and humid should sodium be added to your diet.

Chapter 10

Step 8
Fruits and Vegetables

To change your habits in fruit and vegetable buying start to readjust your thinking. An example of wrong thinking is given by one mother who would buy small, half-rotten apples because they were cheaper but the apples weren't eaten by her children because they were not desirable. How much money did she save by not buying high quality apples her family could enjoy?

Another mother felt that to buy fresh lettuce was too expensive, yet she thought nothing of spending the same amount of money on two cans of green beans. The beans had less nutrition and could be used for fewer meals than the lettuce, so was she right to feel that she was saving money?

To begin with what are the facts on buying fruits and vegetables? Commercially canned fruits and vegetables can be phased out because up to 84 percent of their nutrition is lost in processing. Also, chemicals are often added to retard color changes and stabilize texture. Use the canned goods you have on hand with the thought that they need not be replaced although you can improve the commercially canned fruit you already have by placing it in a colander and rinsing well to remove most of the sugary syrup.

Frozen and fresh fruits and vegetables are better for you than canned fruits and vegetables and when they are purchased in season they are not more expensive.

The following list includes the peak season when each fruit and vegetable is available. The nutrient content of each is also listed.

Apples—available all year; peak October-March; fairly good source of thiamine and minor source of calcium, phosphorus, potassium and vitamins A and C.

Apricots—peak June and July; excellent source of vitamin A and potassium, also contain calcium, phosphorus, and vitamin C.

Artichokes—peak April and May; good source of vitamins A, B_1 and riboflavin.

Asparagus—Mid-February-June; good source of vitamin A.

Bananas—all year; very good source of potassium and vitamin A, fair source calcium, phosphorus, iron and vitamin C.

Beets—all year; peak June-August; good source vitamins A, B_1 and riboflavin.

Blueberries—June-September; good source iron and manganese, small amount of vitamins A and C, calcium, phosphorus and potassium.

Broccoli—all year; peak October-May; excellent source of vitamins A, B and C, rich in potassium, calcium, sulfur and iron.

Brussels Sprouts—peak October; excellent source of vitamins C, B_1 and A, rich in potassium and sulfur.

Cabbage—all year; good source of vitamins C and B_2, rich in phosphorus, magnesium and potassium.

Cantaloupe—May through September; good source of vitamins C and A.

Carrots—all year; excellent source of vitamins A, B_1 and riboflavin.

Cauliflower—September-January; excellent source of vitamins C, B_1 and riboflavin, good source phosphorus, magnesium, potassium, calcium and sulfur.

Celery—all year; good source of vitamins A, B_1, riboflavin, calcium and phosphorus.

Cherries—May-August; good source of vitamin A, iron, copper and manganese.

Corn—early May-September; good source of vitamin A, thiamine, riboflavin, niacin, phosphorus, magnesium, iron and copper.

Cucumber—plentiful all summer; good source vitamin B_1 and riboflavin.

Egg Plant—late summer, July on; excellent source of riboflavin, good source of vitamin B_1.

Grapefruit—all year, most plentiful January-May; vitamin C, small amount calcium, phosphorus, potassium; pink has five times as much vitamin A as the white.

Grapes—July-October; small amount vitamin A, potassium, calcium and phosphorus.

Green Beans—May-October; good source vitamins A, C and B_1.

Lemons—all year; excellent source vitamin C, small amounts of calcium, phosphorus, potassium and vitamin A.

Lettuce—all year; darker-leaf varieties contain six times the vitamin A and three times the vitamin C content than the light varieties.

Limes—all year, peak June-July; same as lemons.

Mushrooms—all year, low in August; good source of thiamine and riboflavin, rich in potassium, phosphorus, copper and iron.

Nectarines—June-September; excellent source of vitamin A, good source vitamin C and potassium.

Okra—peak June-September; adequate vitamins A and C, calcium, phosphorus, potassium and magnesium.

Oranges—all year, peak December-June; good source vitamins A and C, potassium, phosphorus and calcium.

Onions—all year, peak June-September; good source of calcium, phosphorus, potassium and sulfur.

Peaches—June-September; excellent source of vitamin A, good source of niacin, potassium and fair source of vitamin C.

Pears—August-November; low in vitamins A, C and minerals.

Peas—March-June; small amount protein, excellent source of vitamin A, good source of vitamin C, thiamine, riboflavin, niacin, calcium, phosphorus, iron and potassium.

Peppers—most plentiful late summer; excellent source vitamins A and C, also supply calcium, phosphorus, sodium and potassium.

Pineapples—March-June, most plentiful April and May; good source of vitamin C and potassium.

Plums—June-September; dark yellow pulp good source of vitamin A, high in potassium, calcium and iron.

Potatoes—all year; good source vitamin C, niacin, iron, potassium and phosphorus.

Radishes—plentiful all summer; good source vitamin C, calcium, iron, sodium, phosphorus, sulfur, and potassium.

Raspberries and Blackberries—June-August; good source of vitamin A and potassium, fair source of calcium, phosphorus and vitamin C.

Rhubarb—January-June; contains vitamin A, thiamine, niacin, vitamin C, calcium, iron, phosphorus, and potassium.

Spinach—July-November; excellent source of vitamins A, C, riboflavin and potassium; good source of calcium and iron.

Strawberries—peak May and June; excellent source of vitamin C, good source vitamin A, calcium, phosphorus, iron and potassium.

Summer Squash—March-September; good source of vitamin A, potassium, phosphorus and calcium, small amount of vitamin C.

Sweet Potatoes and Yams—all year, peak March-June; outstanding source of vitamin A, also supplies vitamin C, sodium, phosphorus, potassium and calcium.

Tangerines—peak November-January; excellent source vitamin C, good source vitamin A and potassium.

Tomatoes—available all year, peak July-September; excellent source vitamins A and C, also contains calcium, phosphorus, potassium and sodium.

Watermelons—peak June-August; contain vitamins A, C, thiamine, riboflavin, niacin, calcium, iron, phosphorus and potassium.

Winter Squash—October-late winter; excellent source vitamin A, also supplies calcium, phosphorus and potassium.

A complete list of fruits and vegetables to be purchased in the peak season is found in the Grocery Ideas section of this book.

Too many times nutritional value of food is lost in its preparation, but if you follow ideas given here you will preserve those nutrients:

1. Eat vegetables raw whenever possible.

2. Carrots are an exception because they contain more vitamins when cooked. Wash carrots thoroughly but never peel them. Peeling removes precious vitamins close to the carrot's surface.

3. Use a steamer to cook vegetables. If you don't have a steamer simmer your vegetables, but don't boil. To simmer or steam helps retard vitamin loss. And don't overcook. Soft, mushy vegetables lose vitamin content, and they lose flavor as well.

4. Water should be brought to a boil before adding vegetables. Cover the pan tightly.

5. Store cooked vegetables in the refrigerator covered with a lid to retard vitamin loss.

6. Drop frozen vegetables into boiling water while still frozen. Vitamin C is lost during thawing process.

7. Cut carrots and other vegetables lengthwise. Fewer nutrients will escape.

8. Potatoes should be eaten with the skins left on. The potato skin contains 20 percent of the potato's nutrients. Baked potatoes may be eaten skin and all. Potato skins eaten in soups, left on scalloped potatoes or baked with meat will taste better than you may think. Mashed potatoes lose many vitamins in the water as they are cooked. If mashed potatoes must be served, cook in a small amount of water. After cooking, pour left-over water into the blender. Add a small amount of powdered milk and blend. Then pour the milk back over the potatoes and mash.

9. Leave peels on fruits as appropriate. The peels contain many precious vitamins and minerals.

10. Prepare lettuce salads just before serving. Salads prepared ahead of time lose some of their nutritional value.

11. Lettuce should be torn. Cutting causes vitamin loss.

To can and freeze your own fresh fruits and vegetables is an excellent idea. If you do not grow your own, then to buy from a local garden or farmer's market is best. Be sure to choose fresh, firm fruits and young, tender vegetables. Can or freeze the fruits and vegetables as soon as possible after they ripen to ensure a quality product. Purchase a good book or use your local library to find a book with the latest information on canning and freezing.

Consider a food dehydrator to dry your own food. If money for a dehydrator is a problem, make fruit leather (p. 132). This is done by blending the fruit in a blender and letting the resulting puree dry in the sun. If you use your oven for drying, keep the temperature between 120°F to 150°F with the door open slightly. One advantage of fruit leather is that nutritional values multiply in the dried fruit. But if your weight is a problem, remember calories also multiply.

If your children don't like vegetables, let them eat those fruits which are highest in vitamin content. In fact, it's best to always offer good nutritious food from which children may choose. This will make them less apt to rebel.

As you set goals in fruit and vegetable buying, remember it takes time to change your thinking. Each goal, set and completed one at a time, will help you achieve your desired results.

Chapter 11

Step 9
Fruit Juices and Water

Fruit Juices

What drink do you think is the most popular drink in America? If you guessed soda pop, you are right. Millions of bottles and cans of soda pop are bought every day. It would be surprising to many if they were to make a pile of all the soda cans and bottles they emptied in one year. This might well give people the desire to cut down their soda pop consumption.

In a recent newspaper article entitled "Colas Nurture Caffeine Addiction in Kids," Cora Kurty, a nutritionist at the University of Miami, reported that a person may not be aware they are addicted until they drink soda pop without caffeine.[16] She says that a person thus addicted will actually go through withdrawal—suffering headaches, upset stomach and cold sweats.

A report in the *Fort Lauderdale News* compared the caffeine content in nine popular colas. Caffeine measured in a 12-ounce serving ranged from 64.7 milligrams in Coca-Cola to 37.7 milligrams in Diet Rite.[17]

Fruit juices made from 100 percent fruit can replace soda pop. Frozen concentrated orange juice is a favored breakfast drink, but orange juice may be enjoyed anytime during the day. In fact, the many stresses which we endure require more vitamin C for our bodies. Orange juice is a better choice than the artifically flavored powdered drink and they are equally simple to mix.

Fruit drinks in fancy cans and containers do not always contain 100 percent fruit juice. Often, what you are buying is colored water with sugar, artificial flavor added to perhaps only 10 percent fruit juice.

---

16. "Colas Nurture Caffeine Addiction in Kids," *Fort Wayne Journal-Gazette,* October 7, 1979, p. 18A.

17. *Ibid.*

During the winter when citrus fruits are plentiful, fresh-squeezed orange or grapefruit juice is superb. Unsweetened frozen concentrate is also excellent but check what you buy. Frozen orange juice from Florida contains 45 milligrams of vitamin C per 100 grams of juice. Fresh orange juice from California contains 60 milligrams of vitamin C per 100 grams of juice. And beware of pasteurized orange juice. Vitamin C is mostly destroyed during this process.

You may think a popular orange-flavored powdered drink would be a good storage item for emergencies. However, manufacturers fool many consumers with the word "natural."[18] The only natural ingredient in most orange powdered drink is the water. In some areas, even the water would be questionable. Read labels. Learn what is actually going into your body as you drink this "natural" powder.

Unsweetened grape, apple, pineapple, grapefruit and tomato juice are all refreshing and very tasty fruit juices. Prune juice is, in addition, a good laxative.

Carrot juice is high in vitamin A and it has a very sweet flavor. If children start to drink carrot juice when they are young they will probably develop a taste for it. And don't forget V-8 juice—a good blend of vegetables.

Put these natural juices in your pantry instead of soda. They will disappear as you and your family get thirsty for a good drink. When you really want something to quench your thirst, drink nature's water.

Water

The single most important item in our diet is water. It is possible to live as long as five weeks without food, yet only a few days without water.

Even though we see our body of flesh as being solid, it is actually more than 70 percent water since every cell is surrounded and bathed in water.[19]

The minimum amount of water our bodies need each day depends on how much the kidneys need to clear themselves of the by-products of metabolism secreted in the urine. Experts suggest we take into our body three quarts of water a day. This means we need to drink about seven to eight 12-ounce glasses of water daily. Some of the liquid is made by the body itself in the process of breaking foods down. The rest can come from liquids and solid foods.

18. Jane E. Brody, "Don't Take that Natural Food Tag for Granted," *The Ledger-Star,* January 2, 1980, p. 1C.
19. William H. Gregory and Edward H. Goldman, *Biological Science,* p. 509.

Many foods such as watermelon, tomatoes, lettuce, strawberries and even bread contain large amounts of water which add up to your seven glasses of liquid a day. Thus when you combine food, milk and natural juices you will have achieved the proper intake of water to master the second part of Step 9.

Water is so important to the very existence of life that it must be stored for emergencies. Our Civil Defense authorities recommend storing a two-week supply of water which would include one-half gallon per person for drinking and food preparation. Additional water will be needed for brushing teeth, washing dishes, bathing and for use in many other ways.

Store water in heavy plastic containers and add two drops household bleach before capping. If glass containers are used they can be filled with clean water, then processed for twenty minutes in boiling water. In either case, remember that water stored for a long period can lose oxygen, so plan to aerate each container at regular intervals. This can be done by simply turning the container or shaking until bubbles appear.

People who have soft water available in their homes enjoy far cleaner laundry and dishes than do people without soft water. However, soft water for drinking is not recommended since it contains sodium (salt) which your body doesn't need nor is it good for those with high blood pressure. And hard water offers the bonus of a higher mineral content. Some people are able to purchase bottled water which is not necessary, but a nice luxury to enjoy.

Water is 100 percent calorie free—the only liquid or food that is.

Chapter 12

Step 10
Brown Rice

People often think that good nutrition means eating unusual foods that could not possibly taste appealing. "Good nutrition," may bring to mind odd foods such as sea weed, tofu, or miso. Perhaps you put brown rice in this category but brown rice is tasty and may well be preferred over traditional white rice.

Brown rice is rice as it grows. White rice has been "polished" by food processors. This polishing strips the rice of most of its nutritive content including protein and B vitamins. On the other hand, brown rice is a good source of B vitamins and vitamin E and it contains six times as much protein as does the processed white rice.

Use brown rice as you would use any rice. The long grain brown rice may be used for casseroles and main dishes. Short grain brown rice may be preferred for puddings and custards since it is mushier.

To cook brown rice add one cup brown rice and one teaspoon sea salt to two and one-half cups cold water. Bring this to a boil. Boil for five minutes. Cover tightly and simmer for forty-five minutes without lifting the lid. Turn off the heat and let it sit on the hot burner for ten minutes. The rice continues to become tender while sitting the extra time. This amount will serve four people.

If your family doesn't like the taste of brown rice at first, encourage them to try it several more times. Soon they should prefer the nutritious brown rice over the less nutritious white rice.

Chapter 13

Step 11
Syrup and Molasses

Your grandmother bought the "famous brand" syrup, so your mother bought the same brand. You were lucky because when you bought this famous syrup, 2 percent real butter had been added. Lucky? Wrong!

Let's look at the ingredients you poured over your "enriched" white-flour pancakes, or if you are working on Step 2, using whole-wheat, you could be pouring imitation syrup over your honest-to-goodness whole-wheat pancakes.

Did you read the label on the syrup you bought? You might have read: corn syrup 75.2 percent, sugar syrup 20.8 percent, maple sugar syrup 2.0 percent, corn syrup solids, cellulose gum, natural and artificial flavors, sodium benzoate, sorbic acid (preservative) and caramel color.

Many brands of artificial maple syrup are sold in supermarkets, but to use pure syrup from the sap of the maple tree or to make your own honey syrup is preferred. Use honey, a little water and vanilla or maple extract. One mother stretches her maple syrup by adding a little honey. These syrups should all be refrigerated.

More and more supermarkets now carry pure maple syrup. Read the label. Be sure you are getting pure maple syrup. Don't let pictures and the word "natural" fool you. In fact, whenever you fail to read food labels you are missing a great deal of free education.

Even though pure maple syrup is not the cheapest sweet-tooth substitute, it certainly is one of the best. As your tastes change, you can use a smaller amount of this syrup when you serve pancakes.

Quality is more important than quantity. And why does maple syrup have more quality? Maple trees are tapped in March and April. The sap runs down the tree trunk when the nights are cold and days are warm. Maple farmers set a bucket to catch the sap which has no flavor as it comes from the tree since it's mostly water. The farmer boils down the sap which concentrates the sugar and minerals in the sap. None of the minerals are lost during the boiling-down process as the flavorless syrup turns into the yummy, tangy taste we know as maple syrup—a food that is 100 percent natural, untouched by chemicals, unflavored by synthetics and undyed.

You may find that you are cleaning the breakfast table many mornings from excess pancake syrup left all over the plates. Maybe it is better on the plate than in you. What you are cleaning up is a water-base mixture full of sucrose, corn sweeteners, flavored with imitation maple flavoring, dyed with a coal tar dye. Yuk! No wonder your kids now beg for pancakes, waffles, or French toast for breakfast every morning after you started cutting down on sugar and cereals with sugar.

Let us compare white sugar to maple syrup:

100 grams of:	White Sugar	Maple Syrup
Calcium	0	143mg
Phosphorus	0	11mg
Potassium	3mg	242mg
Iron	0.1mg	1.4mg

With these comparisons, the value of maple syrup as compared to white sugar becomes apparent. That many children are lacking calcium is one of Dr. Lendon Smith's complaints in his book *Feed Your Kids Right*. And the nutrition certainly makes maple syrup a better buy. Further, since it is naturally sweet it can be used sparingly so that a little good becomes better than a lot of not so good. Maple syrup not only tastes delicious on whole-wheat hot cakes but it is great used on sweet potatoes and carrots and it makes yogurt into a treat you can enjoy.

Shop around. Compare prices. You can often save over fifty cents a bottle to buy the same amount of maple syrup. Some food co-ops sell it by the gallon. Maple syrup really can help you overcome withdrawal symptoms as you cut down on white, brown and powdered sugar.

Blackstrap molasses is another good sweetener which is full of calcium, iron, B vitamins and other nutrients. Knowing this should make you appreciate the molasses in spite of its taste which is certainly stronger than honey. However, the taste is rarely noticeable when used in baking and cooking. When you serve your next batch of whole-wheat pancakes or cracked-wheat cereal, try putting blackstrap molasses on the table. Children may eventually prefer it to honey on their cereal. It makes the milk look chocolate-y. Besides. it's nice to have a change, so set your goals to include changes to enjoy the flavor of pure maple syrup and blackstrap molasses.

Chapter 14

Step 12
Dairy Products

Milk

Milk is the first food you received as a baby. While milk is not the perfect food, it comes close.

Milk is strong in some nutrients, weak in others. Milk contains nutritionally superior protein. It has all the amino acids essential for the body. It also supplies vitamins A, D, E, and K and the B vitamins. Calcium and phosphorus are also abundant although milk is weak in vitamin C, iron and copper. Unless there is an allergy to milk, it should be included in everyone's daily diet.

Homogenized milk should be avoided. The process of pasteurization turns raw milk from a living food into a dead one. The process destroys all the enzymes and at least 50 percent of the other nutrients. Certified raw milk is acceptable, but it may be hard to find.

Cultured milk is best because the enzymes are already broken down which makes digestion easier. Buttermilk and yogurt are both cultured milks. In fact, buttermilk or watered-down yogurt may be substituted for milk in most recipes.

Powdered milk is good to have in your food storage because it stores well, but store it in an air-tight container in a cool, dry place, and rotate so it doesn't spoil. Non-instant powdered milk has more protein than has the instant. The non-instant contains 16 grams of protein in one cup compared to 8 grams in the instant. Add extra powder to obtain extra nutrition when mixing your milk.

Buttermilk

Buttermilk is so easy to make at home and so economical you will wonder why you didn't make it before. Nor does homemade buttermilk contain additives or preservatives. Buttermilk is a good cultured milk. Buttermilk can be substituted for milk in most recipes. To make your own, take one-half cup buttermilk purchased from the store to add to one quart of milk. (This may be reconstituted powdered milk.) Let this mixture stand at room temperature until it has thickened. Shake or stir before using. Save one-half cup for the next batch. A new start of buttermilk from the store will have to be bought after three or four times.

You will find this homemade buttermilk to be yummier than what is purchased in the store and at less expense, too.

Cheese

Cheese has been around for some four thousand years. Legend has it that an Arab traveled across the desert with milk in a pouch made of a sheep's stomach and by the time evening arrived the milk had separated into part liquid and part solid. The solid the Arab ate as the first cheese.

Cheese is a very good protein. It contains all eight essential amino acids. Try to find natural cheeses which contain the enzymes. Processed cheeses are more expensive in the long run. Processing also involves the use of emulsifiers, preservatives, artificial colors and flavors, chemicals and high heat, all of which affect nutritional value. Milk used to make processed cheese is often milk too old to be sold for drinking.

White cheeses such as Monterey Jack, Swiss or Mozzarella are preferable because of the lack of coloring. Some cheese makers use natural berry juices to color the cheese. Check to discover what you are purchasing.

How can you spot processed cheeses? They are usually in crocks, tins and jars, or they are wrapped in individual slices. Find the natural cheese which best suits you and your family's taste and enjoy the nutritional value.

Cottage Cheese

If hard times should come and you had to depend on your food storage, how nice it would be to know how to make your own cottage cheese. Using only powdered milk from your food storage, you can serve fresh cottage cheese to your family. Combine two and two-thirds cups of powdered milk with seven and one-half cups of water. Stir in one-half cup of buttermilk. Cover this with cloth, not making it airtight. Let this stand overnight until it has clabbered. Heat this mixture very slowly over low heat for up to one hour. Test the curds for cheese-like consistency by pressing the curd between thumb and finger. When the curd stays without slipping away, the cheese is ready. Place in a piece of cheesecloth and let the whey drain off. Salt may be added if desired. Cottage cheese should be refrigerated for future use. Also, look for old-fashioned cottage cheese without preservatives or additives when you buy it from a store.

Butter

A good natural food high in vitamins is butter. Butter has been around for at least the last five thousand years, but only as a food in the last few hundred years.

Margarine is artificially saturated by hydrogenation. Most of the nutrients are destroyed in this process. If any margarine is used, the kind found in a squeeze bottle is preferrable because it has a much lower degree of hydrogenation, but it still contains additives and preservatives.

Unsalted butter eaten in small amounts is better for you than margarine but while butter does contain some essential fatty acids, unrefined cooking oil is preferred for baking and frying. These oils contain more essential fatty acids. To enrich your butter with more fatty acids set out to room temperature then blend with one pound of butter and one cup of soy, safflower or peanut oil. Mold this mixture in a used margarine tub to store in the refrigerator.

Butter helps improve the flavor of foods, satisfy the appetite and stimulate the bile flow. Butter may be enjoyed in moderation.

Eggs

For centuries, eggs have been considered to be highly nutritious. Yet in the last few years egg consumption has drastically decreased because of the cholesterol scare. Many people avoid eggs for fear they will raise their cholesterol level. They believe cholesterol in their blood comes directly from what they eat but most cholesterol does not.

Your body manufactures 80 percent of the cholesterol in your blood through the liver and other organs which leaves only 20 percent of the cholesterol to come from the food you eat. The liver makes more cholesterol naturally than is obtained from foods.

Too much cholesterol in the body may be related to a lack of proper nutrients. Lecithin, vitamin C and grain and vegetable fiber all help to regulate cholesterol levels. Eggs are especially high in lecithin which helps to dissolve cholesterol.

Further, eggs are the number-one protein food. They are an excellent source of vitamin A. Eggs also contain vitamins D, E, some vitamin K, and minerals. Eat at least one egg a day or two if you like. Remember that advertising which encourage you to give up eggs is nearly always based on half-truths.

The fresher the eggs eaten the better. If you have a source where you can get fertile eggs from a farm or eggs from a chicken which was actually allowed to hunt and peck this source is best.

To hard or soft-cook eggs, gently simmer. Hard-cooked eggs should simmer ten minutes; soft-cooked eggs should be left in the simmering water for three to four and one-half minutes. Boiling destroys nutrients; eggs should be simmered. Place cooked eggs in cold water to make peeling easier.

Eggs may be prepared in many different ways—hard- and soft-cooked, scrambled, fried in a small amount of safflower oil, poached, deviled, made into omelets and souffles. Be creative. Enjoy nutritious eggs in your daily diet.

Ice Cream

Ice cream is a treat and should be just that—a real treat not eaten every day. A special occasion is made more special by serving treats such as ice cream.

Beware of ice cream brands which cost less because they are whipped full of air so that you actually get less for your money. The milk used in less costly ice cream is often rejected for sale for drinking purposes because it is too old. Avoid brands with additives or preservatives indicated on the label. Even though all-natural brands cost more, it is better to get a quality product. Remember that all-natural brands still contain high amounts of sugar.

If you want to cut back on sugar, make your own ice cream (p. 133) using a little honey to replace the sugar. Then you can be certain ingredients used are fresh and wholesome. Homemade ice cream can be enjoyed as often as you like because it is not only better for you, but fun for the family to make.

Chapter 15

Step 13
Yogurt

No one can claim to know all there is to know about nutrition because new discoveries are made every day. Maybe you have already made the miraculous discovery of yogurt.

The use of yogurt goes far back in time. The method of preparing yogurt appears to have been passed from one generation to another as an inheritance.

In France there is a legend concerning Emperor Francis, the First. During his reign in the 16th century, the Emperor became gravely ill. Court doctors used their remedies to no avail, then one of them told of a doctor in Constantinople who had a "secret" medicine said to cure ailments such as the one which afflicted the monarch. The doctor was found. His remedy, made from goat's milk, cured the emperor. Since that time, yogurt has been known in France as "la ville eternelle" . . . milk of eternal life.

Persian tradition claims that an angel revealed the method of preparing yogurt to the prophet Abraham. The Persians believe that it was to this food he owed his fruitfulness and longevity.

Today, yogurt is prepared much as it was in ancient times. Warm milk is inoculated with certain health-giving bacteria, then kept warm while the bacteria increase which makes the milk a different consistency. Many people who can't drink milk can eat yogurt. The lack of the lactose enzyme in one's system can cause a milk intolerance and an allergy to milk which can result in an upset stomach. In yogurt, the changes that have taken place in the milk make the lactose enzyme unnecessary.

It is indeed a small miracle how yogurt helps both those who suffer from diarrhea and those who suffer from constipation. Yogurt establishes a well-balanced content for the colon so that neither of these two problems will prevail. Yogurt also helps those who suffer from gas in their stomachs.

Not only is yogurt a good source of protein, it also contains valuable vitamins. In one cup of plain yogurt, there will be:

120 calories
8 grams of protein
295 milligrams of calcium
0.1 milligrams of iron

170 units of vitamin A
0.09 milligrams of vitamin B_1
0.43 milligrams of vitamin B_2
0.2 milligrams of niacin

The calcium in yogurt is already dissolved and therefore more easily absorbed by the body than in fresh milk.

Introduce your family to yogurt—a product which also contains a friendly bacteria, lactobacillus, which aids digestion.

There are many brands of yogurt from which to choose. You may select one which has little or no sugar or additives or you can buy plain yogurt and add your own fresh fruit and honey. Brands which contain sugary preserves should be shunned except for transitional purposes when you can buy fruit-flavored yogurt to help you develop a taste for the product. Many nutritionists recommend eating at least two tablespoons of yogurt a day, but it is great for lunch and yogurt can also take place of the commercial ice cream in your own yogurt pops (p. 135).

Many doctors recommend eating yogurt while at least two of the more common antibiotics, penicillin and ampicillin are taken because antibiotics destroy all intestinal bacteria, even the healthful kind. Yogurt helps to replace friendly bacteria your body needs to fight harmful bacteria.

As you start to enjoy yogurt you may wish to make your own to help you save money and if you make your own yogurt, you have a sure guarantee of pure ingredients. Commercial yogurt is dated on the container but you still have no way of knowing how long it has been on the shelf and active bacteria decreases gradually with time. So the fresher the yogurt the better!

Actually, yogurt almost prepares itself. You can make it in minutes and compare the cost of homemade yogurt at about ten cents per cup as compared to an average of sixty cents per cup for commercial yogurt.

An expensive yogurt maker is not necessary. You need only milk and yogurt "culture" which you can buy at a health food store or you can use yogurt from a good brand of plain yogurt. Once you have started to make yogurt save some from each batch to "start" the next. A fresh start will need to be used after about three or four times.

You will need several plastic containers or empty glass peanut butter jars with tight-fitting lids, an inexpensive candy thermometer and a sauce pan. Also, you will need a box with a lid large enough to hold the plastic containers or jars with small blankets or towels to be used on the inside of the box.

Step 1—Place 2½ cups of water in a sauce pan. Heat to 115° (barely warm to a finger dipped in the water).

Step 2—Use blender to mix 1½ cups powdered milk in warmed water.

Step 3—Add 2 tablespoons plain yogurt. Mix thoroughly. Pour liquid into plastic containers or jars.

Step 4—Cover each container. Place a small blanket or towel on the bottom of the box. Put containers in the lidded box. (Containers may be stacked.) Cover completely with another small blanket or towel. Close the box and put it where it won't be disturbed before processing time is over.

Your yogurt will be ready in three to twelve hours. After it has set, keep it in the refrigerator.

This recipe makes three cups of yogurt. This recipe may be doubled or tripled. The procedure for making yogurt with a yogurt maker is similar. Simply follow manufacturer's directions.

Eat yogurt for lunch or for dinner; eat it between meals when you want a light snack and turn plain yogurt into a nutritious treat in many different ways. Add:

1. Apples (dried or sliced with cinnamon)
2. Bananas (mashed or sliced)
3. Blackberries or blueberries
4. Dates
5. Grape Nuts
6. Granola (homemade)
7. Orange juice concentrate
8. Peaches
9. Pineapple (canned in unsweetened juice)
10. Pure vanilla and honey
11. Raspberries
12. Strawberries (all fruit fresh or frozen)

And any of the above additions can be sweetened with a little honey or pure maple syrup.

Yogurt can be substituted for sour cream or buttermilk in recipes. Try creamy, smooth-textured yogurt on a baked potato. It is yummy, and has fewer calories than sour cream.

Cream cheese can be made from yogurt. Simply place yogurt in a piece of cheese cloth. Tie the ends together. Hang this above your sink to let the whey separate. After about one day of dripping, you will have a smooth, solid piece of cream cheese. Use it as you would use regular cream cheese.

Learn to enjoy the elegance of yogurt. Benefit from its healthful qualities. Start right now to reap the benefits of this "Milk of eternal life."

Chapter 16

Step 14
Unrefined Oils

Visualize in your mind a can of shortening. Do you think of this commodity as health-promoting? Would you eat two tablespoons of this shortening? Nutritionists often recommend two tablespoons of safflower oil to relieve symptoms from such ailments as eczema but there is a difference between safflower oil and solid shortening bought in a can.

Fatty acids are an essential nutrient. Too few people realize that these fatty acids are not derived from many cooking oils and shortenings. Unrefined vegetable oils do contain the essential fatty acids necessary for good nutrition. Safflower oil and sunflower oil should replace saturated oils. Peanut oil and soybean oil may be used for frying or sauteing. These oils should be refrigerated so they will not go rancid.

Most cooking oils are made by heating the grains, beans or seeds. These are then pressed. Further processing results in the loss of vitamin E. Since refined oils lose their nutritional value they are not a good source of unsaturated fatty acids.

Shortening that is solid at room temperature should be phased out because these are hydrogenated, saturated fats. They are hard on the heart, blood vessels and the figure.

Most Americans consume far too many refined oils which contain fat and little else. While your body does need fat, it doesn't need the kind found in refined oils and shortening.

The consumption of too many fats is being proven to contribute to obesity which is a risk factor for heart disease. There are approximately seventy-nine million American adults who are overweight who should realize that unnecessary fats in their diet add extra calories. If these calories are not burned up, they accumulate as fat which will show up on weighing scales. This fat is stored in the thighs, buttocks, and abdomen and soon begins to accumulate around the heart and other vital organs.

Replacing refined oils with unrefined oils will provide your body with essential fatty acids, especially linoleic acid. Two table-spoons of safflower oil, sunflower oil, peanut oil or soybean oil can be obtained daily through salad dressings, mayonnaise or fried foods. When frying food use lower temperatures to avoid the destruction of vitamin E in the oil.

Each time a recipe calls for shortening or vegetable oil, safflower oil or sunflower oil should be used. Adding unrefined oils to your diet can help in assimilation and absorption of the vitamins and minerals your body needs. Reliance upon unrefined oils can prove to be a basic asset to your family's health, heart and happiness.

Chapter 17

Step 15
Homemade Condiments

There are those who may think that it is too much trouble to make their own condiments. After all, mayonnaise, salad dressings, mustard, catsup and vinegar are easily purchased at the store.

Proverbs, chapter 31, gives a report on the qualities of a virtuous woman. In verse 27, we read, "She looketh well to the ways of her household, and eateth not of the bread of idleness." Why would making homemade condiments be looking after "the ways of her household"? How will these homemade condiments benefit a family?

Even though making your own condiments will take more time, consider the advantages to be gained by not giving your "household" the extra additives and preservatives which are found in the commercial condiments.

We have all been given a mind with which to think and reason. Many people depend on the government to protect them from harmful substances. Yet how many times has the government failed? There are cases of many different drugs which have been removed from the market because of harmful side effects. Even birth defects have resulted when an expectant mother takes certain drugs during pregnancy. Your own common sense will help you make decisions.

You may think a small amount of preservatives will not harm you, but do you realize that the average person consumes approximately eight pounds of preservatives and additives each year? Specific harm caused by these preservatives and additives has not been proven, but why wait for harmful effects? Avoid foods which contain additives and/or preservatives.

Mayonnaise

Store-bought mayonnaise is heavily processed. It has been refined, bleached and filtered. Its oils may be "winterized" to keep it from solidifying when refrigerated. This results in the loss of the valuable vitamin E.

See that your family gets all the benefits to be found in mayonnaise by making the easy blender recipe (p. 129). To use your own cold-pressed safflower oil will ensure that you are getting plenty of vitamin E without the preservatives of commercial mayonnaise. Besides being better for you, homemade mayonnaise costs less.

Salad Dressing

When you make your own salad dressing (p. 128) you can free it of preservatives and sugar, and by using your own cold-pressed safflower oil you can be sure you are getting essential fatty acids plus vitamin E.

Most types of salad dressing may be made at home. Use your own unsaturated oil and sweeten with a little honey and you will have nutritious salad dressings to benefit your health.

Mustard

You will benefit by making your own mustard because you will know exactly what you are serving your family. Mustard may be made by mixing vinegar, water and mustard powder together. Place the mustard powder in a bowl and add enough vinegar and hot water to make a paste the consistency of prepared mustard.

Catsup

Homemade catsup (p. 128) need not contain sugar. Only good-quality ingredients need go into your catsup. Your year's supply should be made at the end of summer when tomatoes are plentiful.

Vinegar

Use apple-cider vinegar. White distilled vinegar has few of the naturally occurring nutrients such as potassium so use apple-cider vinegar which has.

In the fall, consider making your own apple-cider vinegar. When you can, freeze, or juice your apples, save the skins and cores. Put these "wastes" into a wide-mouth jar. Add cold water so that the wastes are covered at all times with liquid. Cover with nylon net to keep bugs or flies out.

Keep the jar in a warm place. Add fresh peelings or bruised apples from time to time. When the vinegar smells and tastes strong enough, skim off the top which has thickened. Strain the vinegar and bottle it.

Seeing to your family's nutritional needs and going the extra mile to prepare quality food is worthwhile. Benefits of health are in store for you and your family when you take extra time to prepare homemade condiments.

Chapter 18

Step 16
Chocolate Versus Carob

Well-informed people will agree that carob and chocolate look alike and perform many of the same purposes in creative cooking. Both come from the seeds or beans of a tree. Both are eaten regularly in American homes. But though they have many similarities, they also have important differences.

Chocolate

Chocolate is made from the cacao bean. In Mayan the word cacao means "bitter juice." The beans are fermented and then dried in heat to prevent mold. The beans are then shipped to manufacturers in large bags. The manufacturer cleans, roasts, hulls, blends and grinds the beans. Even though the broken-up beans are quite dry after grinding, they still contain about 54 percent cocoa butter which accounts for the bean's natural fat. When bean fragments are ground finer, the cocoa butter inside is released which forms a substance known as chocolate liquor. All chocolate products are made from this chocolate liquor. Chocolate liquor, whole milk solids and white sugar are the basic ingredients used to make milk chocolate.

The two alkaloids found in chocolate are theobromine and caffeine. An alkaloid is any group of organic bases containing nitrogen found in plants. Even small amounts of alkaloids can have a powerful effect on the body. Medicines and poisons are made from many different alkaloids because of their ability to effect the body's system. Their medicinal values include codeine and morphine used for pain. These alkaloids come from the poppy plant. The alkaloid of the tobacco plant is nicotine which is poisonous to humans. The theobromine and caffeine found in chocolate and cocoa act as stimulants to the nervous system.

The Food and Drug Administration reports that eight ounces of chocolate candy contain 160 milligrams of caffeine, which is 50 milligrams more than a "stay-awake" pill has and which also amounts to nearly twice as much caffeine as there is in a cup of coffee.[20] New findings prove that caffeine is harmful to a fetus.[21]

Oxalic acid is also found in chocolate which has a tendency to combine with calcium when being digested and that means the mineral is unavailable for absorption. Children who are given chocolate or chocolate milk frequently could be losing a considerable amount of needed calcium.

To indulge occasionally in chocolate or cocoa may be harmless, but to eat this food often and in large amounts is undesirable and can become habit-forming. One family who tried living on their present food supply for two weeks reported that the item they missed most was chocolate.

Many hospitals will not take an EEG if a person has ingested chocolate within the previous twenty-four hours. Apparently the caffeine in chocolate disturbs brain wave patterns while affecting the nervous system.

With this information, decide for yourself how much chocolate you want to put into your body. You may find carob to be a delightful substitute.

Carob

The carob tree resembles an apple tree. Carob is also known as "St. John's Bread." There are those who believe that pods and seeds from the carob tree were used as locust which nourished St. John in the wilderness. The dry pods are believed to be the "husks" which provided food for the Prodigal Son. The tree was well known during ancient times. In fact, seeds were so valuable in trade that the word "carat," used by jewelers, comes from the word "carob."

The seeds are very valuable as food. Carob flour is rich in taste and can be compared to the finest chocolate. It does not contain harmful alkaloids, acids, or caffeine and carob is a high-protein food which is scientifically classified as a member of the legume (pea) family.

Carob has a sweet taste because it is 46 percent natural sugar. It also contains B vitamins, especially niacin, as well as calcium, magnesium, potassium and valuable trace minerals. Carob is an especially good source of iron and it is not an empty-calorie food.

---

20. "Caffeine," FDA Fact Sheet, (FDA) 72-3003.
21. "Pregnant Women are Warned by FDA to Avoid Caffeine," The Wall Street Journal, September 5, 1980, p. 32.

Carob can be sweetened with a little honey, molasses, or pure maple syrup in a drink, or to make cakes, cookies or candy. Carob powder, flour and chips are found in health food stores and many supermarkets. With none of the disadvantages of chocolate, carob still has a great taste. The amount you use in recipes will depend on your family's "chocolate-y" taste buds. You will use less honey or sugar with carob than you would use with cocoa.

Hot carob makes a good drink before bedtime. Add a little pure vanilla to wake up the flavor. Or you can make carob chip cookies (p. 130). If you have never tried carob, buy some this week.

Chapter 19

Step 17
Gardening

A back-yard garden can help stretch the food dollar. Berry bushes, grapevines, fruit trees and home-grown vegetables are now gracing the yards of many people. Even though the primary motive may be to save money, do you realize the benefits to be gained by growing more nutritious foods in your own soil? Farmers may be growing crops in soil that is so worn out that nutrients are not available for the proper development of vegetables or fruit. If you grow your own you can be assured of nutrients through proper soil checks.

If space is limited, plant tomatoes or zucchini in the flower beds. Fruit trees fit nicely in any landscape. For those who live in apartments, perhaps an empty lot could be tended by several families together.

A very wise and experienced gardener, Dale White of Fort Wayne, Indiana, has helped many catch the vision of gardening. He shares answers to these often-asked questions as well as sharing his personal gardening techniques.*

Q. I would like to garden, but it seems to be so much work and time consuming. What can I do?

A. Learn to garden the chaise-lounge method. It becomes enjoyable and even profitable. But how do you do this? By mulching the entire garden. Mulch with straw, hay, crushed corn cobs, saw dust, grass clippings, or bark chips. (Do not use grass clippings for two or three mowings if you have applied weed killers to the lawn.) Mulches not only keep the weeds down, but conserve moisture and adds humas to the soil. In fact, if you leave the mulch on the year round, then next spring you will not even have to plow. Just pull the mulch aside and plant. This is a break, isn't it? Also, when gardening by the chaise-lounge method you will need a small table to hold the pitcher of lemonade (made with honey, of course).

---

*Used with permission.

Q. How can I tell when my soil is ready to plant in the spring?

A. One of the most common mistakes gardeners make is working the ground when it is too wet. The best way to tell when the soil is ready is to make a ball of soil and drop it from about three feet. If the ball holds together, it is too wet and you will damage your soil. If the ball breaks apart, it is dry enough to work.

Q. What is meant by intensive gardening?

A. This includes several things: (1) Learn the likes and dislikes of each vegetable. Then plant accordingly. For example, lettuce enjoys cool weather, so plant it beside the tall tomatoes or in the shade of the corn. This is using and conserving space. What flower is more beautiful than the bloom of the eggplant? So, if your garden is small, put an eggplant or two in the flower garden. Is there a plant more frilly than a carrot? Carrots make a beautiful border if you are crowded for room. (2) It also means as soon as one vegetable is harvested, then plant another one in its place. Also, learning when and what to plant for a fall garden and what vegetables can be left in the garden all winter is part of intensive gardening. In other words, learn to make the soil work for you twelve months out of the year, not just a few brief months in the summer.

Q. I have a small garden. What can I grow to my best advantage?

A. There are many vegetables you can grow on a trellis or fence to help conserve space. For example, cucumber, pole beans, and cantaloupe can be tied with silk hose to keep them from breaking loose from the vines. Nylon hosiery is used because it will stretch. Grow tomatoes in cages. Do not let them sprawl. (Do not be mislead by climbing tomatoes or strawberries, there is no such thing.) But you said small. How small is small? Did you know you can feed a family of four the vitamins and minerals they need on a garden plot 20' × 20'? This is why it is good to order from seed catalogs, not the corner grocery store. Seed catalogs will give the growing habits of each vegetable. One year, my sister gave me some squash seed saying they were delicious, but did not tell me how much they grew. I planted them. They grew across the garden, across my strawberry bed, across the alley, across the neighbor's yard and on to her back porch. I was rather embarrassed when she came out and caught me carrying squash from her back steps.

Q. My zucchini grew wonderfully last year, but about the time they started to bloom they died overnight. What was wrong?

A. The squash vine bore did you in. After it hatches from the egg, it enters the squash at the base of the stem. Then it makes a right turn and starts up the center of the stem. If you see the plant start to wilt, check at the base of the plant for some sawdust-like substance. Split the stem until you come to the vine borer. After destroying him, mound dirt up over your slit and the vine will heal.

Q. My cabbage is always riddled with holes and the heads are useless. What is eating my cabbage?

A. The cabbage leaf worm is attacking your cabbage. There are two things you might do: (1) Hire the children to catch all the little white butterflies they see fluttering over your garden. These butterflies lay eggs on the cabbage which hatch into the cabbage worms. (2) You can spray the cabbage and your garden about twice a month with an insecticide. There are two things you can use which are harmless to man, Rotenone and Pyrethrum. The first is ground up roots of a tree grown in South America and Africa. The later is from the mums in your garden. Both are death to bugs, but are not toxic to man. Always spray late in the evening when the bees are in their hives.

Q. Which should I plant, everbearing or June-bearing strawberries?

A. That depends on your desires. Both plants will produce about the same amount of berries. The everbearing will take from spring to fall to do it though. If you wish to put up some for winter, plant the June-bearing strawberries. These produce all at once and stop, while the everbearing put out a few berries in the spring and a few later in the summer and then again in the fall. Berries should produce about one quart per foot of row.

Q. I planted two rows of corn 50 feet long, but got very few ears. What went wrong?

A. There was poor pollination. You should have planted four rows 25 feet long. Corn should always be planted in a block, if possible. The tassel of the corn is the male spores, the silk the female. If the wind happens to be blowing in one direction, it blows the male spores to the neighbor's corn, not yours. If you can not plant in a block, but only a single row or two, then make sure it gets pollinated by going out and cutting off a tassel or two and shake it over the silks of the corn. This is a good experiment for the children. Get a tassel from someone who has red corn and a tassel from your yellow corn. Let them shake some of the pollen from each on the silks. Then put a sack over the ear so no other pollen can produce. You will have speckled corn which is red and yellow. Make gardening interesting for the children. Tell them the necessity of having male and female blossoms and how bees get down into the blossoms. The bees then tromp around thus causing melons, cucumbers, etc., to form. It is an excellent way to teach children their first lesson on sex with no embarrassment to either parent or child.

Q. I had acres of cucumber vines, but very few cucumbers. What did I do wrong?

A. You did not do anything wrong; it was the bees that did not do anything right. That is, unless you planted Gynoecious (all female). It is good to plant some strong smelling flowers in the garden or close by to attract the bees. Sometime, while you are gardening in your chaise-lounge, count the ways bees are depended upon to give us fruits and vegetables. Again you can pollinate your own cucumber if you do not see any bees around. Let the children do some anyway. The blossoms you find with a small pickle growing behind them are female blossoms. Look for blossoms without the small pickle. Peel off the petals and rub some of the spores of the petal into the female blossom. Or, a cotton swab could be used.

Q. I think my cantaloupe crossed with my cucumber this year. They tasted terrible. How can I avoid this in the future?

A. No matter what you hear or what someone tells you, cucumbers and cantaloupe cannot cross. What happened was the weather turned cool and cloudy about the time the cantaloupes were ripening. Sugar is the last thing that leaves the pulp to go into the melons. It takes warm sunny days for the leaves to produce it. So if the weather is unsuited for the process, the cantaloupe will be less than desirable.

Q. I have only a small plot for fruit trees. What can I plant for best advantage?

A. First, that depends on the likes of the family. Apples are always a favorite so plant two apple trees of the same variety. You need two trees to pollinate the apples. Golden delicious are an exception. They will pollinate themselves. Peaches are always a favorite. They will pollinate themselves, too, so one will do. Then you have your choice of plum, cherry, or pear to add to the group. Find which trees grow best in your climate. Then be on the lookout for insects and diseases. They can kill in short order. Do not settle for cheap trees. Why not a grape vine? They are easy to grow and produce well. Plant them on the north side of the garden so they will not shade the vegetables.

Q. Last year I tried growing potatoes, but all I harvested were marbles. What did I do wrong?

A. This, of course, can be caused by lack of fertilizer. Potatoes are heavy feeders so fertilize before planting. Then again right after blossom fall. But I imagine your problem was that you planted too many eyes to the hill. Remember, if you want large potatoes, plant one eye to the hill. If you want large to medium potatoes, plant two eyes to the hill. If you want small potatoes plant three or more to the hill. If you want to grow potatoes and not work weeding or digging, then plant them on top of the ground and cover with ten inches of straw or hay. Then in the fall rake off the hay and pick up the potatoes. If you do not want to get out of the chaise-lounge, tell the kids to pick them up.

Q. How can I keep my carrots from having split roots?

A. The carrot bed must be loose and free of stones. Also, grow shorter carrots. Do not try to grow the long ones you see in the supermarkets for they are often grown in artificial earth that is loose and free of obstruction. Again, you need a seed catalogue that tells the differences and shows the sizes of each.

Q. My family loves cauliflower, but I cannot seem to grow it. What am I doing wrong?

A. Join the crowd. Cauliflower and broccoli both enjoy cool weather in order to produce heads. Try growing it as a fall crop, it is much easier. Let it head up during the cool fall nights in September and October. You can grow the purple head cauliflower which is much easier to grow. The only difference is that the heads are purple and turn green when cooked. Tastes the same, only you need to get used to the color.

Q. How can I keep rabbits out of the garden?

A. Lion dung spread around the perimeter of the garden is supposed to keep them out. You might hire the children to keep them out, but that would cause them to be up all night for that is when the rabbits come. A good 12-gauge shotgun will help. If you choose this method, I can send a good rabbit stew recipe. You could fence in the garden with chicken wire about two feet high. What I am trying to say, it is difficult to keep them out. Just plant some for them.

Q. I have some fruit trees that do not seem to want to bear. They are four to five years old. What is wrong?

A. If they are the full-size trees, they require two to three years more to produce fruit. What you might do is put the trees under stress. This often triggers them to bear. Place a large stone in one of the forks of the tree or tie the branches down. I tied a cord to the branches of my peach tree and pulled them down about parallel to the ground and fastened them to a stake in the ground. The tree bore fruit the first year. Protect the branches with cloth so the cord will not grow into the limb.

Q. I always have lots of seeds left over after planting the garden. Can these be kept until next spring?

A. Yes. Place the seeds in an air-tight jar and store in the re-frigerator or freezer. Many seeds keep their viability for several years, except for celery seeds.

Q. If I should decide to garden the chaise-lounge method, what kind should I get?

A. The kind of chaise-lounge is not important, only that it is comfortable and light, for you will need to get up occasionally to move it into the shade, along with the lemonade.

Try it. You will like it!!!

Gladys Cross, a friend, commented on how uplifting it is to watch her plants grow each week. Her family has drawn closer together as they plant, tend and harvest their garden. Fresh, nutritious fruits and vegetables are now available to her through much of the summer and she has plenty left for canning and freezing. She often says how grateful she is to be able to grow her own nutritious fruits and vegetables.

Chapter 20

Step 18
Nuts, Seeds and Sprouting

Nuts

Squirrels enjoy the flavor of nuts and so can your family. You may think nuts are too expensive but they are actually a good buy for your food dollar because they contain more protein than any other food in the vegetable kingdom. Butternut is 29 percent protein; black walnut is 27 percent protein. Compare this to 22 percent protein in beef. Further, almonds contain all eight essential amino acids and are especially good to use when dieting.

Nuts are high in fat but they are also rich in linoleic acid which is one of the unsaturated fats found to be helpful in regulating cholesterol in the body. Nuts are also a good bargain for your food dollar because they satisfy hunger better by staying in the stomach longer than do most foods.

Many nuts require shelling, skin removal, roasting or simply cutting into pieces. A fun family activity can be learning how to open a coconut. First, pierce the "eyes" with a large nail to drain the liquid from the coconut. To remove the shell easily, put the coconut in a 350-degree oven for twenty to thirty minutes or in the freezer for one hour. While you are waiting to remove the shell, your family could stir up No-Bake Peanut Butter Cookies (p. 133) and your own fresh coconut can then be shredded in which to roll your cookies.

After removing the coconut from the oven or freezer, place on a hard surface. Tap the shell lightly with a hammer until it cracks. Separate the meat from the shell by prying with a strong knife. Shred the coconut pieces with a grater. Roll each No-bake Peanut Butter Cookie in the shredded coconut.

Nuts in food storage should be left in the shell because they retain high quality longer than do shelled nuts, and won't become rancid as quickly. Shelled nuts will keep fresh for several months stored in tightly closed containers in the refrigerator or freezer.

You need to know what food processors have done to nuts. Too many modern processing methods destroy the nutritional value of nuts as they are dyed, bleached and treated with acids and chemicals before they are put into plastic bags, glass jars or cans where their B vitamins rapidly disappear.[22] They are roasted until vitamins are destroyed. They are so heavily salted that their natural flavor is disguised. Nuts in their natural state are a much better food because of their good nutritional value.

There are many delightful ways to serve nuts:

1. As snacks.

2. Sprinkle over yogurt or serve on baked potatoes.

3. Stir nuts into waffle, muffin or biscuit mixture before adding the liquid.

4. Try nuts in tossed salads.

5. Top a vegetable dish with nuts or include in the vegetable dish. For instance, green beans and sliced almonds are a delicious duo.

Seeds

Seeds come in many varieties. The most common seed-forms eaten are sunflower, pumpkin and sesame. These little seeds are packed with nutrition. Other varieties can be used for sprouting.

Sunflower seeds are about 30 percent protein. They are also good sources of phosphorus, calcium, iron, fluorine, iodine, potassium, magnesium, zinc, several B vitamins, vitamin E and vitamin D. Sunflower seeds are also full of magnesium which is the mineral that will enable you to "see the sunny side of life." If you start to feel down, instead of eating a candy bar nibble on sunflower seeds. They can work wonders to brighten a gloomy disposition.

When you buy sunflower seeds purchase only the raw, unprocessed seeds. Sunflower seeds toasted will have lost 90 percent of their nutrition in the process.

Pumpkin seeds are full of minerals. They can be eaten as snacks or ground into meal for baking and cooking. Next Halloween save the seeds for a treat after your jack-o'-lantern has been carved. Roast the seeds in a 350-degree oven. Serve lightly salted or plain.

Sesame seeds are 45 percent protein and they are also an excellent source of calcium, magnesium, niacin and vitamins A and E. The unhulled variety is the best buy since most of the minerals are in the hull. Sesame seeds are used mostly in baking such as in breads, but they can be eaten as a snack.

---

22. J. I. Rodale, *The Complete Book of Food and Nutrition,* pp. 268-269.

Sprouting

Sprouts rival meat for protein. They have more vitamin C than tomatoes and they contain almost all the nutrients your body needs. The sprouting of the seed increases nutritive content of vitamin A by 300 percent and vitamin C by 500 percent. The sprouting process converts starches to simple sugars, which makes sprouts more easily digested than the seeds from which they come.

You don't need a garden to grow sprouts. You can grow them right under your kitchen sink or in any other dark place. Sprouts can be produced very easily with little preparation and they provide fresh vegetables all year.

Alfalfa, mung beans, wheat, sunflower, lentils, rye berries, Alaska peas, sesame seeds and various beans such as lima, soy or pinto are all wise choices for sprouting.

The sprouting of seeds is a very simple process. Cover one tablespoon of seeds with lukewarm water in a pint jar. Do not use chlorinated water because it will kill the sprouts. Let the jar stand overnight. Next morning, tie with string or use a rubber band to secure a piece of cheese cloth or nylon stocking over the mouth of the jar. A canning jar and ring cap can be used to keep the cloth in place. Drain the water into a glass to be used to mix fruit juice or powdered milk for extra nutrition. Turn the jar upside down so the moisture can drain off. The seeds will need to be rinsed two or three times a day. Shake the seeds apart each time you rinse so they won't grow in a tight clump. After three or four days, the seeds will be ready to eat. Eat everything in the jar—old seed, shell, root system, the leaves. Store the covered sprouts in your refrigerator.

Add these sprouts to soups, salads, bread and casseroles just before serving to ensure nutritive content, but keep in mind that sprouts need to be added to bread, meat loaves, casseroles and other baked dishes before cooking. Cut up sprouts if you have to disguise them for particular eaters. And why not try alfalfa sprouts on a sandwich instead of lettuce?

The day may very well come when you will have to depend on sprouts to survive. Develop a taste for sprouts and learn to enjoy their flavor now. Reap the rewards of better health by using sprouts in all your food preparations.

Chapter 21

Step 19
Herbs

Grandma used herbs almost every day to season her foods. Herbs such as basil, oregano, dill, rosemary and thyme bring out the flavor of foods and add variety to your cooking. Herbs can be used to replace salt in your cooking—thyme is especially good.

For centuries herbs have been used for medicinal purposes. There are more than eighty herb drinks from which to choose and most of these are caffeine-free. (There are also herbs which are harmful.)

Good herb drinks for your family to enjoy are camomile, peppermint, spearmint, papayamint, dandelion root and lemon grass— all are available in health food stores.

Herb drinks are a good substitute for coffee, tea and cola drinks. These drinks all contain caffeine which abuse nerve cells. The use of caffeine can also lead to nervousness, insomnia and a lower blood sugar level.

Speaking of bad habits to be broken, there are two others which are harmful to the body. Alcohol has a damaging effect on the human liver. Not only is there the risk of cirrhosis, but alcohol uses up B vitamins and is harmful to the nervous system. The best approach to alcohol is to avoid it altogether.

Even without the surgeon general's warning, common sense would dictate that smoking is hazardous. Use of tobacco in any form is not advisable. It uses up vitamin C in the body. It not only contributes to lung cancer, but is bad for the heart, functioning of the brain, the eyes, nervous system, blood pressure and pulse.

If you desire to use herbs as a medicine, a thorough study of their uses should be made. Then, in consultation with a nutritionally oriented doctor, the principles you learn can be applied.

Herbs may be used to strengthen the body in cases of certain minor illness, but they should be used with judgment.

Chapter 22

Step 20
Vitamins, Food Supplements

The body, like a skillful chemist, is able to correct many of its malfunctions as long as it has the proper chemicals with which to work. Just as you would not take your car to a mechanic without proper tools, you would not expect your body's chemist to fulfill its functions without proper chemicals. Vitamins and minerals are these chemicals.

There are two types of vitamins: fat soluble and water soluble. The four fat soluble vitamins A, D, E and K are found in fatty foods such as cream, butter, vegetable oils and the fat of meat and fish. One characteristic of these vitamins is stability; they are stable when heated so that vitamins are less likely to be lost in the cooking and processing of foods. Other characteristics of these vitamins are that they are not soluble in water nor are they excreted in the urine. Instead, they are stored mainly in the liver.

Water soluble vitamins include vitamin C and the B-complex family. They do not store as well in the body and excesses are excreted through the urine. However, they are absorbed much more easily than are the fat soluble vitamins because they do not rely upon the presence of adequate bile. They are carried by water and they are needed by the body daily. New findings are made every day on the function and importance of vitamins and minerals to our health.

There is, however, much controversy concerning vitamins. There are those who feel that synthetic vitamins (man-made from chemicals) are no different from natural vitamins. Others feel that natural vitamins are best because they are taken directly from living foods. Still others feel they don't need to take vitamins as long as they eat properly.

But there are several reasons why a natural vitamin supplement should be taken:

1. We don't know which farmers are replenishing their soil with proper nutrients before planting.

2. We don't know how pesticides might have affected vitamins and minerals of plants which are our food sources.

3. Our bodies require extra vitamins because of excessive stresses and pressure to which we may be subjected.

4. Artificial vitamins are made from chemicals in the laboratory, and do not give the same results.[23] Natural vitamins come from natural food sources.

Just as it is impossible to match mothers milk in a laboratory, it is also unlikely that a synthetic vitamin can be a duplicate that is equal in quality to a natural vitamin. They might look the same and might even trigger our bodies chemistry to react in similar ways but natural is best.

Did you know that in many cases vitamin C can be substituted for a decongestant; that children who have leg pains and experience loss of hair need more vitamin C in their diet? Have you heard that the mineral calcium has been known to reduce and to relieve pain from menstrual cramps and "charlie horses"? Did anyone ever tell you that after they started taking B-complex vitamins they noticed an improvement in their patience and emotions? Did you know that taking an adequate amount of B-complex vitamins can even relieve morning sickness for many expectant mothers? Have you heard about the remarkable recovery of those who take vitamin E after experiencing a heart attack? There are new findings every day on the function and importance of vitamins and minerals.

Add a good vitamin book to your library to help you understand what your body needs to reach optimum health. Dr. Lendon Smith, a well known pediatrician, has written a book entitled, *Feed Your Kids Right*. This book is a medical dictionary which specifies doses of vitamins and minerals to be taken to aid your body in fighting many common illnesses. If natural vitamins are taken to build up resistance to bacteria and viruses, then large doses will not be required to repair and rebuild sick bodies. Because everyone's body chemistry is different, the amounts of vitamins needed will also be different.

Eat properly, exercise and take those extra vitamins so your body's chemist will have the help needed to bring you to your optimum health.

_____

23. Charles Gerras, *The Complete Book of Vitamins*, p. 41 and 200.

Chapter 23

P.S. And Baby, Too!

Problems can arise when changes are made in the diet of older children. But a newborn baby has formed no diet habits. What better time to begin a good nutrition program for that newborn?

The trend for many years has been to bottle feed babies. Many mothers are now returning to nature's way of breast feeding. Mother's milk is far superior to anything bought in a can. Prepared formulas contain up to 56 percent sugar.

Mothers who desire to give their baby the nutritional advantage of nursing can be successful. A short study of breast feeding before the baby arrives will help prepare the mother. A trip to the library can turn up several good books on the subject.

If breast feeding is not successful choose a formula which is either very low in sugar or sugar free. Sugar does not build bodies. A baby needs protein for growth and development.

A time to start babies on solid foods may vary. After six to eight months, you should be ready to start giving your baby one to ten teaspoons of oatmeal. Sprinkle wheat germ on the cooked cereal and add a small pinch of brewer's yeast, gradually increasing the amount each time. Then your homemade applesauce may be added to the cereal. Make applesauce for the baby by placing one raw peeled and diced apple and one-quarter cup apple juice in the blender. Cottage cheese with equal amounts of pureed fruit may be served to your baby. Carrots or beets, steamed and mashed, can be added next.

Mash bananas with a fork, then add milk, wheat germ, brewer's yeast or tapioca. How convenient to take a banana with you as you travel or when you go out to dinner. Fruits such as peaches or pears may be pureed in the blender with a small amount of orange juice.

After the baby is about nine months old, cooked egg yolk may be added. Avoid the white of the egg for a while because of possible allergy. When the baby is a year old fowl, fish, lamb or veal may be added to the diet. Honey should be avoided for the first year of the baby's life because microorganisms found in honey can be harmful to an infant until their digestive system is sufficiently developed. Also, some studies have associated the use of honey ingested by infants to crib deaths.[24]

To have your child develop a taste for brewer's yeast, yogurt and carrot juice will be to your advantage as the child grows older. Help your baby accept brewer's yeast by adding one-quarter teaspoon. Gradually increase this amount to foods daily. If your baby is bottle-fed, yogurt, which provides valuable intestinal bacteria, may be introduced early into the diet. But since breast milk supports the growth of bacteria within the intestine yogurt can be introduced later. Instead of Kool-Aid or Jello water put carrot juice in the baby's bottle. It's sweet and it will give the baby lots of vitamin A. Unsweetened apple, grape and strained pineapple juice are excellent juices to give the baby, especially when ill. Giving them Kool-Aid or Jello water develops a craving for sugar. It's the clear liquid they need, not the refined sugar.

Feeding your baby need not be complicated nor bothersome and using these food ideas will make feeding your baby pleasantly simple. If a food needs to be heated, place it in a small heat-resistant custard cup and set it in warm water.

With the cutting of more teeth, your baby is ready to eat the same foods you do and a natural liquid supplement will help to ensure that your baby is getting what he needs. Babies are happier when they are receiving the proper foods to keep them healthy. To use these ideas will give you a start toward good nutrition for your baby.

---

24. Patricia Hermes, "WD Medical Update: Crib Death," *Woman's Day*, February 10, 1981, p. 16.

Unit III
Getting Organized

Chapter 24

Goal Selection

As you ponder these principles of good nutrition you may understandably feel overwhelmed with the knowledge that you must revitalize your family's diet. The suggested Twenty Steps to Better Nutrition can help you make these changes. Now set goals. If *you* focus on one step at a time you can accomplish your desires.

Perhaps you are convinced that goal-setting is essential to improve your purpose in life. For instance, to set a goal such as "To become a perfect mother" is unrealistic. Perfection is an on-going process to be attained through developing specific habits in needed areas. Benjamin Franklin exemplified such an approach. He made a list of ten virtues he would like to develop and then worked on each until he had perfected himself in all ten areas.

The same principle will work for you in setting goals for better nutrition. To set one goal at a time will help you concentrate on one step at a time.

Jenny Lee used the following goals to help her get started in the changes she desired to make. Her list will give you an idea of goals to help with your transition program. Write in your own goals as they apply to your family. Have a target date of when you will want each goal completed. As you complete one, the circle can be colored by that goal so that you can see your accomplishments. To observe your progress will give you a sense of satisfaction.

Jenny Lee's Goals

Step 1, Study Nutrition   *Target Date*

O Plan a night with the family to teach good
   principles of good nutrition.   _____

93

O Check out good books from the library. Make
a thorough study of nutrition.   _____
O _____ (Set your own goals in this space.) _____
O _____ _____

Step 2, Whole-wheat
O Purchase wheat for food storage.   _____
O Purchase or borrow a wheat grinder.   _____
O Make homemade bread.   _____
O Serve cracked wheat-cereal, whole-wheat
pancakes and waffles.   _____
O Buy unbleached white flour instead of bleached
white flour.   _____
O Add wheat germ and bran to casseroles
and cereals.   _____
O _____ _____
O _____ _____

Step 3, Cereals
O Use cereals that contain less than 10 percent
sugar.   _____
O Make home-made cereals.   _____
O Serve more whole-wheat pancakes, eggs,
and cracked-wheat cereal for breakfast.   _____
O _____ _____
O _____ _____

Step 4, Junk Food
O Read labels at the grocery store.   _____
O Circle junk foods (Chapter 6) as they are
eliminated from the grocery list.   _____
O Decide which alternative to junk food will
be used.   _____
O Make a grocery list and use it to shop on
grocery day.   _____
O Make a treat from natural ingredients for a
night with the family.   _____
O _____ _____
O _____ _____

Step 5, Honey
O Purchase items in which sugar is listed third
or fourth on the ingredients label.   _____
O Replace small amount of honey for sugar in
baking.   _____

The Church of Jesus Christ of Latter Day Saints
Adrian Ward

March 11, 2018

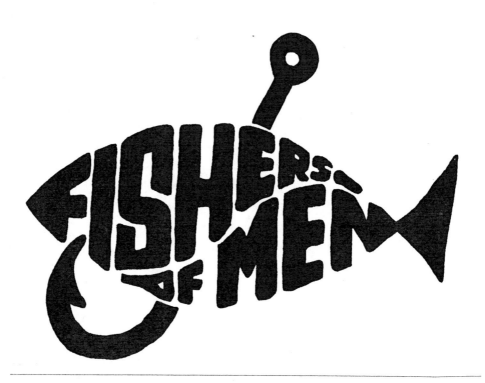

The Church of Jesus Christ
of Latter Day Saints

Presiding..Bishop Marshal Finch

Conducting..Mark Gallup

Chorister.......................................Sister Martha Ellis

Organist...................................Sister Elizabeth Rose

Opening Hymn...#84 Faith of Our Fathers

Invocation...Antonia Rosalez

Ward Business

Sacrament Hymn...#181 Jesus of Nazareth

Administration of the Sacrament

Speaker...Grace Evans

Speaker..Jeannie Majeske

Young Women Vocal
"Peace in Christ" Accompanied by Mckendra Perry

Speaker..David Dyerly

Closing Hymn...#45 Lead Me into Life Eternal

Benediction...Joan Brewer

Bulletin Preparation is done on Wednesday to print Thursday.
To submit bulletin announcements, contact Sister *Pam Purk by either calling 734-279-2930 or by emailing pjpurk@hotmail.com*

To schedule appointments with Bishop Finch, please contact
Brother Tom Majeske at 517-423-2919.

Adrian Missionaries may be reached at 517-442-5999.

Please serve our Missionaries by inviting them for a meal. Sign up either outside the Relief Society Room or by contacting them personally.

Young Women's March Schedule

All activities 6:30-7:30 PM unless otherwise indicated:
14 – SERVICE AND FUN – hymnal repair and MIA Maids will teach group games.
21 – Cake decorating with McKendra Perry 7-8 PM
28 – Combine YM and YW. YM are in charge of program.

REMINDER FOR WARD CLEANING MARCH:

14-17 – Ben & Kalli Nash, Bob & Jill Wessell, Salem Wade
22-24 – Tom & Jeannie Majeske, Barbara Glisson, Katie Hall, Bonnie Draper
Special Instructions: Please contact Sister Heidi Lee if you need access to the building 517-442-2852.

All Sisters please join us for lunch on Wednesday, March 14, 11:30 AM at Papa's Coney Island, corner of US 223 and Treat Highway (on back side of BP gas station) Adrian. No agenda – just eat and chat.

Ann Arbor Stake Single Adult Activity (ages 31 and up), Saturday, March 17, 11 AM to 2 PM at Institute Bldg. 914 Hill Street, Ann Arbor. Bring your favorite board game and enjoy along with pizza, salad and pop. There is also ping pong and billiards. Questions? Contact Sam Gines at sammy500@aol.com

Next **Empty Nesters** will be Saturday, March 24, 4 PM at the Adrian Ward Cultural Hall hosted by Norm and Janet Lichtenberg and Martha Ellis. Only those who are personally contacted to bring something will need to bring a dish to share. PLEASE COME ENJOY GREAT COMPANY, GOOD FOOD AND A FUN TIME. HOPE TO SEE YOU THERE!

Coats and more needed locally! Please donate your **"gently" used** *"adult only"* men's and women's coats, gloves, hats, socks, sweatshirts and blankets. Bring them to the Relief Society Room so they may be donated to the homeless in the Adrian Area. Questions?? Contact Sharon Oelke please. **No children's clothes please!**

If there is anyone in the Adrian Ward either **Vocal or Instrumental Talents**, who would like to perform 'uring our Sacramental Service, please contact Janet Lichtenberg.

The **Lost & Found Box** has been moved to outside of Relief Society Room under the table. Unclaimed items will be donated to charity.

Would you like to volunteer giving back to the community throughout the year? **JUSTSERVE.com** *contact Brother Frank Purk 734-279-2930*

Building Calendar Scheduling contact *Brother Spencer Folau 517-451-9612*

Family History Center hours for the general public are Wednesdays 7-8:30 PM and Thursdays 2-6 PM. Additional hours are by appointment only by calling *Sister Jeannie Majeske 517-423-2919*

The **Ward Library** is available to all teachers for class preparation, all Ward members for talk preparation, family home evening and any other need with which the library may assist. We encourage you to use these resources. **As respect to others, when you borrow any resource, please return it promptly to either that same shelf or file.** The library is open on Sunday and by specific request as prearranged with reasonable notice. If anyone has either a question or would like help with any library materials, contact *Sister Jill Wessel by phone 443-808-5992 or email jsw59kgy@gmail.com*

Please remember our Ward Missionaries while away on their callings:
Elder Dakota Dallin Perry, 1120 Cole Drive. SW, Lilburn, GA 30047
Elder Christian Ammon Folau, Kirche Jesu Christi, Corneliusstrausse 18, 60325 Frankfurt am Main, Germany
or email at **christian.folau@myldsmail.net**
Elder Samuel Finch, Calle Los Agrologos 368, Urbanizacion Las Acacias De Monterrico, La Molina, Lima 12, Peru
Sister Victoria Martinez, 6833 West Bell Road, Glendale, AZ 85308
Sister Carys Bott, Rua Belo Horizonte, 1236 Centro, 86020-061 Londrina – PR, Brazil
Sister Samantha Griffes, 1624 Wanless Drive, Brampton ON L7A 0A7, Canada

Call ahead to schedule your session at the **Detroit Temple** at 248-593-0690 and share a ride by carpooling. *Remember our monthly Ward Trip is on the second Saturday of every month for the 11 AM session.*

O Replace traditional sugar treats with your
   own nutritional treats. Add these recipes to
   recipe file. _____

O _____ _____
O _____ _____

Step 6, Protein

O Count the grams of protein to see if enough
   is obtained in one day. Plan ways to increase
   if necessary. _____

O Plan meals to use less beef. Use half the
   beef called for in a recipe. _____

O Find a source where beef is raised without
   harmones or antibiotics. _____

O Use poultry more often. _____

O Use fish at least once a week. _____

O Avoid pork. (Bacon, lunch meat and hot
   dogs.) _____

O Use dried beans to provide extra protein. _____

O _____ _____
O _____ _____

Step 7, Peanut Butter and Salt

O Buy 100 percent natural peanut butter. _____

O Cut down on salt intake. Use salt only on
   the table or only when cooking. _____

O _____ _____
O _____ _____

Step 8, Fruits and Vegetables

O Phase out all commercially canned fruits
   and vegetables. Can or freeze my own. _____

O Form better food preparation habits to
   save nutrients. _____

O _____ _____
O _____ _____

Step 9, Fruit Juices and Water

O Phase out soda pop and artificially flavored
   drinks. _____

O Use only 100 percent fruit juices. _____

O Drink more water. _____

O Store enough drinking water for a two
   week emergency. _____

O _____ _____
O _____ _____

Step 10, Brown Rice
O Replace white rice with brown rice. _____
O _____ _____
O _____ _____

Step 11, Syrup and Molasses
O Purchase maple syrup for pancakes. _____
O Try molasses in baking. _____
O _____ _____
O _____ _____

Step 12, Dairy Products
O Purchase certified raw milk or non-instant
   powdered milk. _____
O Use cultured milk in baking. _____
O Make buttermilk at home. _____
O Buy natural, unprocessed white cheese. _____
O Make cottage cheese or buy the natural without
   preservatives. _____
O Stretch butter with safflower oil. _____
O Purchase farm-fresh eggs where possible. _____
O Make homemade ice cream for a night with the
   family. _____
O _____ _____
O _____ _____

Step 13, Yogurt
O Learn to enjoy the flavor of yogurt by eating at
   least two tablespoons a day for a week. _____
O Make homemade yogurt to save money. _____
O _____ _____
O _____ _____

Step 14, Unrefined Oils
O Replace shortening with unrefined safflower,
   sunflower, peanut or soybean oil. _____
O _____ _____
O _____ _____

Step 15, Homemade Condiments
O Make homemade mayonnaise. _____
O Make salad dressing using safflower oil. _____
O Prepare mustard from vinegar, water and
   mustard powder. _____
O Make catsup when tomatoes are plentiful. _____
O Use apple-cider vinegar. _____

O _____ _____

O _____ _____

Step 16, Chocolate Versus Carob
O Purchase carob chips and carob powder. _____
O Use one-half chocolate and one-half carob to
gradually cut down on chocolate. _____
O Use carob more to substitute for chocolate. _____
O Make carob chip cookies. _____
O _____ _____
O _____ _____

Step 17, Gardening
O Plan the garden for next spring. _____
O Plant the garden in the spring. _____
O _____ _____
O _____ _____

Step 18, Nuts, Seeds and Sprouting
O Try nuts in different ways to flavor dishes served. _____
O Crack open a coconut for an activity with the
family. _____
O Serve seeds to the family for snacks. _____
O _____ _____
O _____ _____

Step 19, Herbs
O Enjoy herb drinks more often. _____
O Study herbs and their uses. _____
O _____ _____
O _____ _____

Step 20, Vitamins and Food Supplements
O Purchase, and take, good, natural vitamins to
supplement better eating habits. _____
O _____ _____
O _____ _____

To change a life-time of habits will take time. There will be minor setbacks along the way. Overcome these small discouragements and continue your good nutrition program. As each goal becomes a habit, set your next goal.

The following story points out the importance of following guidelines:

Two friends were walking over many country roads. One said to the other, "I am not traveling any special road pattern, yet we are not lost. I have had my eye on the high-tension electric line. It goes to our destination."

The road they were traveling was rutted. It was easy to follow the ruts, but where the sand had blown in they could have been lost yet they weren't. They had kept their eye on their guide above.

Your goals for good nutrition are important. Follow them. They will help you reach your final destination of better health for you and your family. Success will come if you take time to make a plan. To set each goal and reach it is your key to success.

Chapter 25

Menu Planning

To serve nutritious, healthy meals start with menu planning. You may think menu planning is boring and time consuming, but good nutritious meals begin with menu planning which can be both fun and time-saving.

As mentioned earlier, many meals served lack necessary nutrition. Good nutritious meals must be thought out to replace these inadequate meals. The typical American breakfast, described earlier, which consists of white bread with jelly, artificial-imitation orange drink, margarine and imitation eggs must be replaced with wholesome, healthy food. Planning a weekly breakfast menu will help.

First, list all the nutritious breakfasts you can think of that your family would enjoy. Your list will probably include many of the following:

Breakfast Ideas

1. Energy French Toast (p. 118)
2. Whole-wheat pancakes (p. 119)
3. Eggs (poached, hard- or soft-cooked, scrambled, fried)
4. Cracked-wheat cereal (p. 118)
5. Homemade granola (p. 118)
6. Homemade cereals (pp. 117-119)
7. Fried egg sandwich.
8. Hot cereals (old-fashioned rolled oats, millet, soy grits, rye grits).

If your family leaves in the morning without breakfast, they miss the most important meal of the day. Call a family council to see what can be done. Older children can be given the responsibility of starting breakfast when they arise. Suggest breakfast ideas the night before to get a head start. For instance, whole-wheat pancake batter can be prepared then. Refrigerate until morning and stir before using. (If your family won't eat whole-wheat pancakes, try your usual recipe using unbleached white flour fortified with wheat germ and a little brewer's yeast. Then gradually add whole-wheat flour to your mix, increasing the amount each time.)

For those mornings when everyone oversleeps, make a mixture for a vitamin-and-mineral-rich protein drink to be made in the blender. Use soy powder, wheat germ and a little brewer's yeast in milk or fruit juice. Fortify the Orange Julius (p. 133) or the Banana Smoothie (p. 129) recipe with this mixture and serve a real treat for breakfast. This mixture, known as "Instant Protein," may even be bought already combined in a health food store.

Even if you can't cook every morning, you can plan good breakfasts that will be easy and quick. If you don't have a plan, then it's too easy to go back to boxed cereals containing sugar. Easy, quick ideas for breakfast might include:

1. Yogurt with fresh fruit
2. Piece of fresh fruit
3. Whole-wheat toast with honey
4. Hard-cooked egg (previously cooked)
5. Homemade granola with milk
6. Protein drink

Breakfast can include several of these ideas but remember to include high-protein items such as yogurt, milk or eggs to help see you through the day.

Whichever way you choose to go, begin right now to make your menu schedule using a chart similar to the one on page 105 and fill in breakfast ideas your family would like. Remember to consider the total grams of protein as discussed in the protein chapter. Also, take into consideration which mornings you might be more rushed and prepare a simple, quick meal.

This chart can become a permanent part of your kitchen. It may be covered with clear contact paper and taped to the inside of a kitchen cabinet for easy reference. These breakfast menus can be the same each week so that, once planned, no more thought need be given to breakfast planning. If you rise a bit bleary-eyed, how nice it will be to have breakfast already planned.

Now that breakfast is taken care of, it is time for lunch. What are you going to do to replace the inadequate meal of a bologna sandwich on white bread, potato chips, a slice of processed cheese and imitation fruit drink? Make a list of appropriate foods to replace such inadequate meals. Good ideas could include:

1. Tuna salad sandwich (p. 120).
2. Chicken salad sandwich.

3. Egg salad sandwich
4. Cheese spread sandwich (p. 120)
5. Cheese toastie (p. 120)
6. Peanut butter and honey sandwich
7. Broiled chicken pieces
8. Cheese and whole-wheat crackers
9. Tuna and onions with lemon juice
10. Meat loaf sandwich
11. Hard-cooked eggs and cheese
12. Broiled tuna and cheese sandwich (p. 120)

Try to plan a definite lunch menu for each day. Put these lunch ideas on the chart on page 105 to keep inside that kitchen cabinet beside the breakfast chart.

Dessert can come from the snack list but it isn't really necessary to have a gooey sweet every day. Also, as your children come home from school, train them to choose their after-school snack from the snack list.

The following snacks are nutritious, and healthy and much needed for your children's growing bodies. They also will not do you any harm.

1. Peanuts in the shell
2. Sunflower seeds
3. Pumpkin seeds
4. Raisins
5. Celery
6. Carrots
7. Dried fruit
8. Popped wheat
9. Fresh fruit
10. Cheese sticks
11. Popcorn
12. Apple or celery with peanut butter
13. Bell pepper slices

A list of snacks you and your family like can go beside the chart with the breakfast and lunch menus which you keep posted in your kitchen. Also, list treats or desserts your family likes best. To have these ideas posted will make your decisions about what to prepare for snacks or dessert easier.

Many may find the convenience of prepacked dinners tempting because they seem to be easier and quicker. Actually cooking from scratch at home does not take much more time. Several good, quick dinner recipes are included in the recipe section of this book.

To use a monthly menu plan will save time as well as ease the daily agony over what to serve for dinner. As you begin to organize menu ideas, try dividing your menus into beef night, casserole night, fish night, soup night, chicken night, cheese night and Italian-Mexican night, or invent your own night. This can be the same night each week, with only the main dish changed.

A sample chart of all menu ideas is found on page 106. Make your own menu idea chart like the one in this book and fill in your own menu ideas. This chart may then be used to help you make choices as you fill in your monthly menu chart (p. 107). Use the monthly menu chart to plan your monthly menus. The chart can be covered with clear contact paper. Use a crayon or felt-tip pen to fill in main-dish ideas from your menu ideas chart which will then be reusable each month.

As you fill in your main-dish ideas take into consideration more hurried evenings when a soup night would be more welcome. If each day of the week is designated for a specific night this will make your menu planning easier and more organized. As you eat less beef, replace beef night with another idea.

Many recipes you have are already nutritionally adequate. Check the ingredients. Perhaps only a few changes or additions will be necessary to make them more nutritious. The following chart will help you know what changes or additions to make:

Recipe calls for:	Substitute:
Sugar	Honey
Shortening	Safflower oil
Cream of mushroom soup	Cream sauce
White bleached flour	Unbleached white flour plus one-half whole-wheat flour or one-half soy flour
Milk	Buttermilk
Sour cream	Yogurt
Cocoa powder	Carob powder
Chocolate chips	Carob chips

Additions

Wheat germ
Bran
Brewer's yeast
Sunflower seeds
Sesame seeds
Raisins
Extra vegetable (such as carrots to casserole dishes)

Until your family has developed a taste for cookies or cakes made with whole-wheat flour or soy flour, ease the transition by making your own cookies and cakes with unbleached white flour adding wheat-germ and a small amount of brewer's yeast. Wheat germ may be whizzed in the blender to make it so fine no one will be any the wiser.

As you substitute honey for sugar, remember that honey is much sweeter than sugar so use less honey and even less each time the recipe is made. (Recipes using honey may need to be cooked 25 degrees lower, since they might burn more easily.)

Don't be afraid to experiment with a recipe to obtain a more nutritional dish. In fact, experimenting will make your baking more interesting.

After you have filled in your main-dish ideas on the menu chart, select the vegetables and salads you would like to serve with each meal. The following ideas should prove helpful.

Vegetables

As you choose vegetables for your monthly menu chart, remember to choose those which are in season. Use the chart in the grocery section (pp. 112-113) to find which vegetables are in season for the month for which you are planning. Or use vegetables you have canned or frozen yourself.

The following vegetables should be included often because of their high vitamin content:

1. Broccoli
2. Brussels sprouts
3. Carrots
4. Cauliflower
5. Peas
6. Sweet potatoes
7. Tomatoes

Salad

Salads served with each meal can add variety and will also provide adequate nutrients. Your monthly menu chart can include these salad ideas:

1. Peach salad (p. 127)
2. Applesauce (p. 126)
3. Tossed salads (p. 127) (Use a variety of vegetables beyond the standard lettuce and tomatoes. Try different types of darker green lettuce to replace iceberg head lettuce. The darker the green the more vitamin content there is in the lettuce.)
4. Waldorf salad (p. 128)
5. Winter fruit salad (p. 128)
6. Summer fruit salad (p. 127)
7. Carrot salad (p. 126)

8. Pineapple-Banana Boat (p. 127)
9. Mushroom-Broccoli salad (p. 127)

Remember to use fruits in their peak season. Fruits which should be included often because of their high vitamin content are:

1. Apricots
2. Nectarines
3. Peaches
4. Strawberries
5. Tangerines
6. Papaya
7. Melons (canteloupe and watermelon)

Your monthly menu chart can be erased and changed each month or it can be much the same except for necessary changes to allow for fruits and vegetables in season. However you do the charting, it should be according to you and your family's desires and tastes.

As you use these food ideas to replace your inadequate meals, you will find how easy menu planning is. You will actually save time by being prepared each month.

BREAKFAST MENU

Sunday	Monday	Tuesday	Wednesday	Thursday	Friday	Saturday
Homemade Granola	Eggs poached scrambled hard-cooked	Hot cereal	French toast	Bulgar or Cracked-wheat	Pancakes or Waffles	Fried egg sandwich
Toast	Toast	Toast	Yogurt	Toast	Yogurt	Milk
Protein fruit drink	Milk	Protein fruit drink		Protein fruit drink		
Juice or Fresh fruit	Juice or Fresh fruit	Juice or Fresh fruit	Juice or Fresh fruit	Juice or Fresh fruit	Juice or Fresh fruit	Juice or Fresh fruit

Lunch Ideas

Tuna and onions
Cheese Toastie
Tuna Salad
Cheese Spread
Peanut butter and honey
Chicken salad
Egg salad
Meat Loaf
Hard-cooked eggs and cheese
Broiled chicken
Homemade soup

Snacks

Peanuts in the shell
Sunflower seeds
Pumpkin seeds
Raisins
Bell peppers
Celery
Carrots
Dried fruit
Popped Wheat
Fresh fruit
Popcorn
Cheese sticks
Apple or celery with peanut butter

Treats

Orange Julius
Banana Smoothie
Yogurt Popsicles
Fruit Bread:
   banana
   zucchinni
   pumpkin
   carrot

MENU IDEAS

Sunday	Monday	Tuesday	Wednesday	Thursday	Friday	Saturday
Beef Night:	*Casseroles:*	*Fish:*	*Soups:*	*Chicken:*	*Cheese:*	*Italian-Mexican:*
Roast	Beef Stroganoff	Poached Fish	Cracked-wheat	Baked	Macaroni and Cheese	Pizza
Round Steak	Fried Rice	Salmon Patties	Potato	Broiled	Grilled Cheese	Tacos
Sirloin Steak	Chow Mein	Tuna Casserole	Chili Con Carne	Chicken a la King	Easy Chicken	Enchiladas
Swiss Steak	Meat Loaf	Fish Casserole	Chicken	Chicken Casserole	Chicken Tetrazzini	Lasagna
Liver			Vegetable			Spaghetti
Beef 'n Noodles			Stew			
			Bean			

MENU CHART

Sunday	Monday	Tuesday	Wednesday	Thursday	Friday	Saturday
Vagetable: Salad: Liver	Meat Loaf	Poached Fish	Chili	Chicken a la King	Macaroni and Cheese	Enchiladas
Roast	Fried Rice	Salmon Patties	Cream of Potato Soup	Broiled Chicken	Easy Chicken Casserole	Pizza
Round, Swiss or Sirloin Steak	Chow Mein	Tuna Casserole	Vegetable Soup	Baked Chicken	Chicken Tetrazzini	Tacos
Beef 'n Noodles	Beef Stroganoff	Fish Casserole	Chicken Soup	Chicken Casserole	Grilled Cheese	Spaghetti

Vegetable Ideas:
1.
2.
3.
4.
5.

Salad Ideas:
1.
2.
3.
4.
5.

Chapter 26

Grocery Ideas

Now that your menus are planned, you are ready to go to the supermarket. To plan grocery purchases will save time in the store and money for your food budget. A grocery list will help curb impulse buying.

Most supermarket managers place their most tempting, tasty treats right in the front of the store. Here you will find goodies or soda pop on sale. How much easier it will be to pass by these with your grocery list clutched firmly in your hand. Your resolve to change your eating habits will be that much stronger when you decide ahead of time what you will buy.

If you decide just what to include on your list and if you buy only these selected items you will have achieved a personal victory. Consider Mary Smith who came home from a grocery trip lasting two hours with only one bag of groceries. Her husband asked, "Where have you been?"

"I've been reading labels at the grocery store."

This was the starting point for Mary Smith because she learned that only by reading ingredient labels could she determine which items to choose. Mary was amazed when she realized that items she had usually purchased were more than half sugar, they were also full of additives and preservatives and they contained few vital foods. She knew that it was time for a change.

And you can change by using the ideas in this book to help you in your grocery purchases. Make a list of foods you want to include:

Produce

1. Apples
2. Bananas
3. Bell peppers
4. Broccoli
5. Carrots
6. Celery
7. Mushrooms
8. Lettuce
9. Onions and garlic
10. Oranges
11. Pineapple
12. Spinach
13. Sweet potatoes
14. Tomatoes
15. White potatoes

108

Dairy Products

1. Butter
2. Buttermilk—remember you can make your own
3. Cheese—preferrably white, unprocessed with the enzymes intact
4. Cottage cheese—natural without additives or make your own
5. Eggs—farm fresh are best!
6. Milk—certified raw or non-instant powdered are preferred
7. Yogurt—plain—to be used for the start of home-made

Meats

1. Fish—fresh or canned are best
   a. Tuna
   b. Salmon
   c. Sardines
2. Chicken or turkey—scout around to see if these are raised locally by someone who feeds them only grains and no chemicals
3. Beef—also try to find a cattle raiser who does not use DES or antibiotics
4. Liver

Frozen Foods

1. Orange juice concentrate
2. 100 percent lemon juice
3. Fruits
4. Vegetables

Miscellaneous

1. Cereals—less than 10 percent sugar for transition; hot cereals—rolled oats for cooking and granola
2. Dried fruits
   a. Dates—read label for unsweetened
   b. Prunes
   c. Mixed dried fruits
   d. Raisins—unsulfurated
3. Fruit juices—no sugar
   a. Apple
   b. Grape
   c. Prune
   d. Tomato
4. Catsup—home-made as soon as possible!
5. Mayonnaise—home-made, now!

6. Peanut butter—natural
7. Pure vanilla extract
8. Salad dressing—make this at home
9. Tomato sauce—homemade, too
10. Spices and herbs
11. Unbleached white four—good for transition

Health Food Store or Co-op

1. Bran
2. Raw wheat-germ
3. Brewer's yeast
4. Sunflower seeds—raw
5. Sesame seeds
6. Seeds for sprouting—alfalfa, mung bean
7. Brown rice
8. Whole-wheat pasta
9. Carob powder
10. Carob chips
11. Soy flour
12. Whole-wheat flour—until a grinder is bought!
13. Safflower oil
14. Honey—buy only raw, unfiltered
15. Nuts
16. Kelp
17. Iodized sea salt
18. Pure maple syrup
19. Molasses
20. Coconut—unsweetened

Your list may be somewhat different, but this will give you an idea what to include when you make up your own list. Each week it will be so easy to look over your own list to jot down what is needed. A list of fruits and vegetables in season is found at the end of this chapter. It can be used when you plan menus for the month.

Shopping in the "L" shape helps to save time and temptation. Most stores are laid out so that produce is along one outside wall while dairy products line the next outside wall. This forms an "L" shape. To confine most of your shopping to this area may save you from "impulse buying." Use the "L" shape to help you walk past aisles filled with convenience foods. There are some 8,000 items in the average supermarket. Limit yourself to view only those certain ones you plan to buy—and this will help in your decisions, decisions, decisions!

A mother who truly desired good health for her children be-moaned, "My daughter eats too much junk food. I don't know what to do." A friend suggested that her daughter couldn't eat junk food unless the mother bought it. She should simply tell the child what the choices are for a snack from the snack list.

Mary Smith found to her pleasure that as she bought fewer junk-foods and more naturally good food, her food dollars stretched farther. Making her own bread. mayonnaise, buttermilk and meals from scratch also helped. If her grocery bill had increased, the extra money would be worth it because she was helping her family build bodies with the foods they ate.

Bad habits have a way of catching up to you. Keep in mind that doctor's visits, allergy shots, hospital stays all cost, too. To put your money into good food for healthier bodies makes more sense.

Here are ways to help you save money in the food store:

1. Always use a list. Buy only what is on the list.

2. Cook from scratch. Avoid convenience foods. Convenience foods can be as much as three times more expensive than are home-made foods.

3. Shop on a full stomach. Gurgles and rumbles from an empty stomach may tempt you to buy something you did not plan to buy.

4. Buy produce in season when it costs less and also tastes best.

5. To buy food storage items in bulk often will lower the over-all price.

When planned for, grocery shopping can be a pleasant expe-rience; one to look forward to as the time when you choose food to promote your sweet family's health.

FRUITS AND VEGETABLES BOUGHT IN SEASON

January	February	March	April	May	June
Apples	Apples	Apples	Artichokes	Artichokes	Apricots
Bananas	Asparagus	Asparagus	Asparagus	Asparagus	Asparagus
Broccoli	Bananas	Bananas	Bananas	Bananas	Bananas
Brussels Sprouts	Broccoli	Broccoli	Broccoli	Broccoli	Beets
Cabbage	Brussels Sprouts	Cabbage	Cabbage	Cabbage	Berries
Carrots	Cabbage	Carrots	Carrots	Cantaloupe	Blueberries
Cauliflower	Carrots	Celery	Celery	Carrots	Cabbage
Celery	Celery	Grapefruit	Grapefruit	Celery	Cantaloupe
Grapefruit	Grapefruit	Lettuce	Lettuce	Cherries	Carrots
Lettuce	Lettuce	Mushrooms	Mushrooms	Corn	Celery
Oranges	Oranges	Peas	Peas	Grapefruit	Cherries
Potatoes	Potatoes	Pineapple	Pineapple	Green Beans	Corn
Rhubarb	Rhubarb	Potatoes	Potatoes	Lettuce	Cucumbers
Sweet Potatoes	Sweet Potatoes	Rhubarb	Rhubarb	Mushrooms	Green Beans
Tangerines		Summer Squash	Summer Squash	Oranges	Lettuce
Winter Squash		Sweet Potatoes	Sweet Potatoes	Peas	Limes
				Pineapple	Mushrooms
				Potatoes	Nectarines
				Rhubarb	Oranges
				Strawberries	Onions
				Summer Squash	Peaches
				Sweet Potatoes	Peas
					Pineapple
					Plums
					Potatoes
					Radishes
					Rhubarb
					Strawberries
					Summer Squash
					Sweet Potatoes
					Watermelon

FRUITS AND VEGETAGLES BOUGHT IN SEASON

July	August	September	October	November	December
Apricots	Bananas	Bananas	Apples	Apples	Apples
Bananas	Beets	Blueberries	Bananas	Bananas	Bananas
Beets	Berries	Cabbage	Broccoli	Broccoli	Broccoli
Berries	Blueberries	Cantaloupe	Brussels Sprouts	Brussels Sprouts	Brussels Sprouts
Blueberries	Cabbage	Carrots	Cabbage	Cabbage	Cabbage
Cabbage	Cantaloupe	Cauliflower	Carrots	Carrots	Carrots
Cantaloupe	Carrots	Celery	Cauliflower	Cauliflower	Cauliflower
Carrots	Celery	Corn	Celery	Celery	Celery
Celery	Cherries	Egg Plant	Grapes	Lettuce	Lettuce
Cherries	Corn	Grapes	Green Beans	Mushrooms	Mushrooms
Corn	Cucumbers	Green Beans	Lettuce	Potatoes	Oranges
Cucumbers	Egg Plant	Lettuce	Mushrooms	Spinach	Potatoes
Egg Plant	Grapes	Mushrooms	Potatoes	Sweet Potatoes	Sweet Potatoes
Grapes	Green Beans	Nectarines	Spinach	Tangerines	Tangerines
Green Beans	Lettuce	Onions	Sweet Potatoes	Winter Squash	Winter Squash
Lettuce	Nectarines	Peaches	Winter Squash		
Mushrooms	Peaches	Peppers			
Nectarines	Peppers	Plums			
Onions	Plums	Potatoes			
Peaches	Potatoes	Spinach			
Peppers	Radishes	Summer Squash			
Plums	Spinach	Sweet Potatoes			
Potatoes	Summer Squash	Tomatoes			
Radishes	Sweet Potatoes				
Spinach	Tomatoes				
Summer Squash	Watermelon				
Sweet Potatoes					
Tomatoes					
Watermelon					

Chapter 27

Baking Day

Baking day can become one of the most enjoyable days of your week. Just to know that time spent making homemade items that will provide for better health to your family will give you great satisfaction.

As you get organized and become familiar with your recipes, baking day will take only a few hours of your morning. Set aside a certain time each week to do your baking. Try to make this a definite time. Be careful not to let other events interfere with your baking schedule. Working women might use part of Saturday morning or an evening to do their baking. Time spent preparing healthy food for your family is time spent ensuring your family's health.

Some mothers may begin better nutritional practices because it saves money. For instance, one mother figured that she could save $708.24 a year by mixing her own non-instant powdered milk and by making her own whole-wheat bread.

Milk, 5 gallons a week

Kind	Price per gallon	Yearly Price
Homogenized	$1.89	$491.40
Instant Non-fat	$1.20	$312.00
Non-instant	$ .44	$114.40

Bread, 7 loaves a week

Kind	Price per loaf	Yearly Price
Store bought wheat	$1.29	$469.56
Homemade	$ .38	$138.32

Savings can be anywhere from $510.64 to $708.24 yearly depending on the type of milk used.*

---

*Food prices vary from region to region. These prices were taken from the West Michigan area.

This price comparison was enough to spur this mother on to spend extra time to bake at home. Only later did she appreciate the nutritional advantages she gained as well.

As you begin your baking day habits, here are helps to get you organized.

1. Start with a clean tidy kitchen. This will make the task seem easier. Clutter can cause frustration.

2. List the items you want to make. This will help you plan your time.

Bread	Cracked Wheat
Syrup (made with honey)	Cream or Cottage Cheese
Yogurt	Buttermilk
Salad Dressing	Grind Wheat Kernels for Flour
Mayonnaise	Pasta
Granola	Sprouts

You may not want to start by making everything on the list, but once you get going, everything will not have to be made each week. For instance, once you have made salad dressing, it should last for several weeks.

3. Write recipes used for baking day on 3 by 5 cards and keep them together. This will save time.

4. Keep ingredients you will use together. Set these on the counter before you start.

5. Have hot dish water in the sink to wash and drain your bowls and utensils. This will save time at the end of your baking.

6. Save salad dressing bottles, mayonnaise jars, etc. in which to store your homemade items.

7. Double recipes as appropriate to your family size.

8. Make enough bread to last one week. Check your oven to see how many loaves can be baked at one time. If your oven will hold six loaves triple your recipe.

9. You will need the appropriate number of loaf pans, a large mixing bowl (you can use a large, round plastic bowl) and a large spoon.

10. If you have never made bread before, start with a single recipe until you feel confident before you double or triple the batter.

11. Many women knead their bread in the bowl. If this is uncomfortable, turn the dough out on a floured surface to be kneaded.

12. Shape dough into loaves immediately after kneading. To let the dough rise twice is really not necessary (unless you plan to enter a bread-making contest.) The dough will be soft and spongy if you use the method described in the recipe section for homemade bread.

13. If you feel it is necessary to let the bread rise twice, then let the dough rise in the same pan in which you mixed it.

14. Your week's supply of bread can be stored in the refrigerator or freezer.

Other Tips on Getting Organized

● Make pancake batter the night before so you don't have to rush so in the morning.

● Hard-cook one dozen eggs after grocery shopping to use for breakfasts, sandwiches, deviled eggs, etc.

● Clean vegetables to be used for snacks during the week and keep them in the refrigerator in a tightly covered container.

List of equipment to make baking easier:

1. Blender
2. Bread maker (make your bread by hand if money is tight)
3. Pasta maker (buy pasta in the health food store until you can make your own)
4. Six bread pans
5. Two large cookie sheets with edges (to be used to make a double recipe of granola)
6. Canning jar with ring lid and piece of nylon stocking or cheesecloth (to be used to start sprouts)
7. Candy thermometer (for yogurt making)
8. Several small containers or peanut better jars with tight fitting lids (for yogurt making)
9. Box with lid and several small blankets or towels (for yogurt making)
10. Steamer (for cooking vegetables)

Anyone can make excuses or rationalize that they don't have time for a baking day. But if you set this as a high priority in your life, you will *make* time to see that your family receives the good wholesome foods they deserve.

Remember that most children love to cook. What a special time to spend together talking and teaching future mothers and fathers.

Chapter 28

Recipes

To help your children avoid the temptations of too much junk food, always have plenty of tempting, nutritious food on hand. Use the following recipes to get off to a good start.

The recipes have been divided into breakfast, lunch, dinner, salad and snacks and dessert sections to make it easier for you to find and to plan. These recipes have all been kitchen tested and found to be favorably accepted. You will definitely become a hit with your loved ones when you serve these tasty morsels.

BREAKFAST RECIPES

Bran Flakes

2 cups bran	½ tsp. sea salt
2 cups whole-wheat flour	¼ cup safflower oil
½ cup dry powdered milk	1 tbsp. molasses
2 tsp. brewer's yeast	1 cup water

Combine all the dry ingredients. Make a well in the center and add the safflower oil, molasses, and water. Mix well. Divide in 3 parts and roll out as thin as possible on greased cookie sheets. Bake 350º for 15 to 20 minutes or until golden brown and crisp. Break into small pieces. Store covered in the refrigerator.

Corn Bread

1 cup yellow cornmeal	½ tsp. sea salt
1 cup whole-wheat flour	1 cup milk
2 tbsp. honey	¼ cup safflower oil
4 tsp. baking powder	1 egg

Oil square 9 x 9-inch pan. Blend all ingredients for about 20 seconds. Beat vigorously for one minute. Pour into pan. Bake at 425° for 20 to 25 minutes.

117

Cracked-Wheat Cereal

1 cup cracked-wheat
1 tsp. sea salt
4 cups water

Method 1: Cook over direct heat for about 30 minutes. Reduce water to 3 cups, if desired. Stir frequently.

Method 2: Cook in double boiler for 1 hour or more.

Method 3: Start in double boiler at night and cook for 30 minutes to 1 hour. Let stand until morning, then cook for at least 30 minutes more.

Energy French Toast

Use desired number of eggs to which you add a small amount of milk and several tablespoons of bran, wheat-germ and a small amount of brewer's yeast. Dip whole-wheat bread slices in mixture and pan fry both sides.

Granola

3 cups rolled oats	½ cup unsweetened coconut
½ cup wheat germ	½ cup sunflower seeds
⅓ cup honey	½ cup almonds
⅓ cup safflower oil	1 cup raisins
	½ cup walnuts

Mix rolled oats, wheat germ, unsweetened coconut, sunflower seeds, nuts, raisins and toss thoroughly. Combine oil and honey. Add to dry ingredients. Mix until crumbly. Pour mixture into shallow baking pan brushed with oil. Place on middle rack of oven. Bake at 300° for 20 minutes, stirring once. Store covered in the refrigerator or freezer.

Oatmeal

Use milk instead of water to make oatmeal. Add one-half cup wheat-germ at the end of cooking before the cereal sets up. Sprinkle with cinnamon.

Transitional Whole-Wheat Bread

1 tbsp. yeast	1 tsp. sea salt
¼ cup warm water	¼ cup safflower oil
2½ cups hot water	3 cups whole-wheat flour
⅓ cup honey	5 cups unbleached white flour

Soften yeast in warm water. Combine hot water, honey, salt and oil. Cool to lukewarm. Stir in whole-wheat flour and 1 cup white flour;

beat well. Stir in yeast. Add enough of remaining flour to make moderately stiff dough. Knead until smooth (10 to 12 minutes). Let rise in same pan as mixed or shape into loaves as desired. Bake at 350° for 40 minutes. Makes two loaves.

Wheat Flakes

1½ cups whole-wheat flour	½ tsp. sea salt
¼ cup wheat germ	¼ cup peanut butter
¼ cup soy flour	

Combine whole-wheat flour, wheat germ, soy flour and salt. Beat peanut butter with water until smooth. Add to dry ingredients to make a soft dough. Add more water if necessary to be able to roll the dough. Roll, and bake at 350° for 15 to 20 minutes. Store covered in the refrigerator.

100 Percent Whole-Wheat Bread

Here is a method for making bread that will be appreciated by harried homemakers and especially by women who work. This bread-making process is started the night before the bread is actually cooked. The evening before you want your finished product, place 2 tablespoons baking yeast, 1 teaspoon honey, and ¼ cup warm water (110°) in a bowl. Allow the yeast to activate. In a larger bowl, put ⅓ cup honey, ⅓ cup safflower oil, 1 tablespoon sea salt and 6 cups warm water or milk. Two eggs can be added at this time. Add 6 cups whole-wheat flour and mix. Add the yeast mixture. Beat about 50 times. This mixture is stored, covered, in the refrigerator overnight to allow the gluten to develop. (If you are making bread the same day, allow this mixture to stand at room temperature for at least four hours.)

The next day (or evening after work) let this mixture stand at room temperature for one hour to warm. Knead in approximately 6 cups of *sifted* whole-wheat flour. Knead for at least ten minutes. Shape into loaves and let rise in the bread pans until double. Cook at 350° for 35 to 40 minutes. This recipe can be doubled or tripled. Yield—4 loaves.

Whole-Wheat Pancakes

1½ cups sifted whole-wheat flour	1½ cups milk
1 tsp. baking powder	3 tbsp. safflower oil
¾ tsp. salt	2 egg whites beaten *stiff*
2 egg yolks	

Combine in order given, folding in beaten egg whites last. Makes 12 very light whole-wheat pancakes.

Yogurt or Cottage Cheese Special

Mix yogurt or cottage cheese with any combination of nuts, seeds, wheat germ, bran or fresh fruit.

LUNCH RECIPES

Cheese Spread

Grate your favorite kind of cheese. Add a small amount of mayonnaise.

Cheese Toastie

Thinly slice cheese. Place on a slice of slightly buttered whole-wheat bread. Place in the broiler until cheese is melted. May use mayonnaise instead of butter if desired.

Toasted Tuna Sandwiches

Drain can of tuna. Add grated cheese, slice hard boiled eggs and/or diced onions. Spread this mixture on wheat buns. Place in the broiler until the cheese is melted.

Tuna Salad

Drain can of tuna. Add chopped apples, celery, onions and small amount of mayonnaise. Spread on whole-wheat bread to make sandwiches.

Tuna and Tomato Salad

    ½ head of lettuce (large)
    2 tomatoes (large)
    1 can of tuna (small)
    2 sticks of celery
    2 large carrots

Toss and add a small amount of homemade mayonnaise.

DINNER RECIPES

Baked Chicken

Wash whole chicken. Place in large, covered pan. Sprinkle with garlic powder. Cook at 500° for 1 hour.

Beef 'N Noodles

Cook small piece of meat such as roast for several hours in small amount of water (enough to cover the meat). Cook until tender. Refrigerate until grease has formed on top. Remove the grease. Shred meat into fine pieces. Heat water until boiling. Add whole-wheat noodles. Cook until noodles are tender (about ten minutes).

Beef Stroganoff

½ pound ground beef
3 cups mushrooms, thinly sliced

¾ cup onions, thinly sliced
1 cup yogurt

Brown meat; drain. In separate pan, saute mushrooms and onions. Add to meat mixture. Add yogurt; heat being careful not to boil. Season with sea salt or kelp. Just before serving add handful of alfalfa sprouts, if desired. May be served over brown rice or whole-wheat noodles.

Cheese Puffs

Make six sandwiches with white cheese slices and whole-wheat bread. Place sandwiches in a 9 x 13 pan. Cover with mixture of 4 eggs (beaten) and 2½ cups milk. Let stand overnight in refrigerator. Bake for 30 minutes at 350°.

Chicken A La King

1 cup mushrooms
½ cup butter
½ cup diced green pepper
½ cup unbleached flour

½ teaspoon sea salt
2 cups milk
1¾ cups chicken broth
2 cups chicken, cooked

In a large skillet, cook mushrooms and green pepper in butter until tender. Blend in flour. Stir in milk and broth. Stir in chicken and serve over brown rice.

Chicken Rice Casserole

Cook brown rice as directed in chapter on brown rice (p. 61). Add 2 to 3 cups cooked chicken and 2 cups white sauce. Heat in 350° oven until warmed. Cheese added to white sauce makes a nice variation.

Chicken Soup

Bring chicken broth to a boil and add any amount of vegetables desired; left over chicken-pieces, whole-wheat noodles or brown rice. Frozen or fresh corn, peas, carrots, celery are good. Cook until tender. Salt and serve hot.

Chicken Tetrazzani

1 cup chicken, cooked
1 cup white sauce

1 cup white cheese, shredded
2 cups cooked whole-wheat spaghetti

Add all ingredients and heat until cheese melts.

Chili Con Carne

2½ cups pinto beans
2 quarts water
1 pound ground beef
2 cloves garlic
1 onion chopped
1 medium green pepper,
  chopped

1 quart whole tomatoes
¾ cup tomato paste
1 cup Savorex (prepared)
3 tbsp. chili powder
  or to taste
2 tbsps. oregano

Soak beans over night in water. Next morning bring to boil and simmer, covered, for one hour. Brown meat, add onion, garlic, green pepper. Drain fat and add tomatoes, tomato paste, Savorex, chili powder, oregano and salt to taste. Cover and simmer for one hour. Add beans and 2½ cups of the cooking liquid to the meat mixture. Cover and simmer for 2 to 3 hours longer.

Cracked-Wheat Soup

1 pound ground beef
1 quart whole tomatoes
1 quart water
1 cup tomato sauce
1 cup water
1 cup carrots

½ cup celery
1 package dry onion soup mix
2 bay leaves
½ tsp. garlic powder
½ cup cracked-wheat
  few sprigs parsley

Brown and drain hamburger. Add remaining ingredients. Bring to a boil. Add cracked wheat. Stir for 2 minutes. Simmer for 30 minutes.

Cream of Potato

4 cups fat skimmed chicken
  broth
2 cups double-strength
  powdered milk, reconstituted
3 tbsp. unbleached white flour
½ cup cold water

potatoes, diced
carrots, diced
fresh mushrooms, if desired

Heat chicken broth to boil. Add potatoes and carrots, bringing to second boil. Lower heat to simmering. Cook until potatoes and carrots are tender. Add reconstituted powdered milk and heat until simmering. Combine water and flour into a smooth paste and stir into the simmering soup until thickened slightly. Add sliced mushrooms and simmer 6 to 8 more minutes.

Chow Mein

½	pound ground beef	2	cups water
1	medium onion, chopped	½	tsp. sea salt
1	cup chopped celery		mushrooms, sliced
3	tbsp. soy sauce		water chestnuts, sliced
2	tsp. Savorex		bamboo shoots
3	tbsp. corn starch		green peppers, sliced
			bean sprouts

Brown the meat. Drain off the grease. Saute celery, onion, mushrooms and green peppers in oil in a separate pan. Add Savorex (similiar to beef broth, but better for you; sold in health food stores) and water to meat mixture. Add soy sauce. Heat to boiling. Blend corn starch and small amount of water to make creamy paste. Add gradually to meat mixture. Add sauted vegetables and remaining ingredients. Heat gently. Serve over brown rice.

Easy Chicken Casserole

1	bunch fresh broccoli or	2	cups cooked chicken
1	package frozen broccoli	2	cups white sauce
2	cups grated cheese		

Cook broccoli until almost tender. Place cut-up broccoli in a large casserole dish. Add the rest of the ingredients and mix thoroughly. Bake in 350° oven for 30 minutes or until it bubbles.

Enchiladas

Soften tortilla shells in 350° oven for 5 minutes. Sprinkle each shell with ¼ cup shredded cheese and heaping tablespoon of onion; roll up. Place in a baking dish. Pour chili (may use left-over chili con carne) over and sprinkle with grated cheese. Cook at 325° for 25 minutes or until it bubbles.

Fish Casserole

2	pounds fish fillets	2	stalks celery, chopped
1	cup fresh mushrooms		parsley, chopped
1	onion, diced		salt
1	cup grated white cheese		paprika

Place the fish in lightly oiled dish. Lightly salt. Layer remaining ingredients except paprika. Sprinkle with paprika. Bake at 350° for 30 minutes. Serves 6.

Fried Rice

Use one cup of cold brown rice (prepared the day before) and one egg per person. Fry two onions, chopped carrots and green peppers in ⅔ tablespoons of oil. Add the rice, stirring with a wooden spoon. After 5 minutes, add the eggs which have been previously beaten with a small amount of milk and flavored with soy sauce. (Make sure your brand of soy sauce is made from soy beans. Some commercial brands of soy sauce are almond-flavored salt water.) Stir until the eggs have set. Small amount of cooked ground beef or left-over chicken is good in this dish.

Grilled Cheese Sandwiches

Place sliced cheese between two slices of whole-wheat bread. Grill on each side in a hot skillet in a small amount of butter.

Liver

Rub liver with lemon juice. Coat the liver in unbleached white flour, paprika and crushed thyme. Saute sliced onions in safflower oil. Set aside to serve as a side dish or to embellish the liver. Heat more oil to cook the liver about 3 minutes on each side.

Macaroni and Cheese

Cook whole-wheat macaroni in boiling water for 10 minutes. Drain and add grated cheese such as mozzarella or Monterey Jack. Add a small amount of milk. This mixture may be heated in a casserole dish in the oven until the cheese has melted.

Meat Loaf

1 pound ground beef	¼ tsp. sage
¼ cup cooked brown rice	¼ cup chopped celery
¼ cup oatmeal	1 egg
¼ cup wheat germ	¼ tsp. sea salt
¼ cup tomato juice	¼ cup chopped onions

Mix all ingredients in a large bowl. Place mixture in oiled pan. Bake at 350° for 45 minutes or until done. Serves 5 to 6.

Pizza Dough

3 cups whole-wheat flour	1 tbsp. yeast
1 tsp. sea salt	¼ cup warm water
1¼ cup milk	3 tbsp. safflower oil
3 tbsp. honey	

(Part of the flour may be unbleached white flour for transitional purposes.) Mix yeast and warm water. Let stand to get a good start. Add honey, oil, milk and 1½ cups flour. Knead for 5 minutes. Add remaining flour and knead 5 minutes more. Let rise 45 minutes to 1 hour. Press into pizza pan. Cover with choice of pizza topping.

Pizza Toppings

1 cup tomato sauce	soy protein bacon-bits
bell pepper	2 cups mozzarella cheese
mushrooms	½ tsp. oregano
onions	

Poached Fish

1 medium onion, sliced	½ tsp. sea salt
1 tbsp. lemon juice	1 bay leaf
3 sprigs parsley	1 pound fish fillets

In a large skillet, heat to boiling 1½ inches water with onion, lemon juice, parsley, bay leaf and salt. Arrange fish in single layer in the skillet. Cover; simmer 6 to 10 minutes or until fish is tender.

Salmon Patties

Drain one can of pink salmon. Mash the bones to give added calcium. Add one or two eggs, whole-wheat crackers or bread crumbs. Make patties and fry until brown on both sides.

Spaghetti

Brown onions and garlic in 1 tablespoon safflower oil. Brown 1 pound ground beef. Drain off grease. Add 3 cups tomato sauce, ½ teaspoon oregano, salt to taste. Simmer for 45 minutes to 1 hour until a thick sauce. Serve over cooked whole-wheat spaghetti.

Stew

Cut a roast into small pieces. (Half a roast could be used and the rest saved for another recipe.) Coat with unbleached white flour and brown in ¼ cup butter in a skillet. Place this in a large pan and cover with water. Simmer for several hours until tender. Add diced potatoes, cubed carrots, chunks of onion, sliced celery, 2 tablespoons parsley, 2 cloves garlic and 2 bay leaves. Simmer for 30 minutes until the vegetables are tender.

Swiss Steak

Brown steak on both sides. Cover with fresh or frozen tomatoes (peeled and mashed) and sliced onions. Cook until tender, about 1½ hours.

Tuna Casserole

Drain one can of tuna. Add cooked whole-wheat noodles and white sauce. Bake 350° for 30 minutes.

Vegetable Soup

Cover a soup bone or a small roast with water in a large pan. Simmer for several hours. Take the meat off the soup bone or cut the roast into small pieces. Add diced potatoes, sliced carrots, small cubes of cabbage, chopped onion, frozen mixed vegetables, 1 teaspoon celery seed, 2 cups tomato juice. Simmer 30 minutes or until done.

White Sauce

  1 tbsp. butter
  1 cup milk
  1 tbsp. unbleached white flour

Melt butter in a sauce-pan. Stir in the flour. Continue to stir until smooth. Gradually add the milk, stirring constantly. Heat until the mixture thickens. Mushrooms could be sauteed in the melted butter to make a mushroom sauce. One cup cheese could be melted in to make a cheese sauce.

SALADS

Applesauce
  4 medium-sized apples   ⅛ cup apple juice
                                   1 tsp. cinnamon

Wash and core the apples. Place all ingredients in the blender to blend.

Carrot Salad

Grate 2 pounds of carrots. Add one can of unsweetened pineapple, 1 cup raisins, small amount of mayonnaise, 1 teaspoon vanilla, a little juice from the pineapple and a little milk. Toss thoroughly.

Cole Slaw

Cut cabbage into small bite-size pieces. Add chopped apples, raisins and small amount of mayonnaise.

Favorite Salad
spinach   avocado
lettuce   onion

Wash spinach and lettuce thoroughly. Add slices of avocado and onion. Serve with your favorite salad dressing.

Mushroom-Broccoli Salad

Cut 1 pound fresh mushrooms and 1 bunch fresh broccoli into small bite-size pieces. Sprinkle with soy protein bacon bits (these may be found in the health food store without sugar) and homemade whole-wheat croutons. (Croutons may be made by cutting slices of whole-wheat bread into cubes. Sprinkle with melted butter and garlic powder. Brown in broiler.) Serve this salad with Creamy Garlic dressing. (Recipe on p. 128.)

Peach Salad

Place peach half on a lettuce leaf. Top with cottage cheese in the pit opening. Decorate with wheat germ or cinnamon.

Pineapple-Banana Boat

Take a fresh pineapple and cut in half length-wise. Cut the pineapple out being careful to leave the shell intact. This shell can be the serving dish with the edges cut in diamond shapes. Fill the shell with cut-up pineapple pieces and sliced bananas. Seedless grapes and sliced strawberries may be added for color and variety.

Summer Fruit Salad

Combine fruits which are in season in the summer such as cherries, grapes, plums, watermelon or cantaloupe. Serve with whipped cream sweetened with a little honey or pure maple syrup.

Tossed Salad Supreme
Combine any of the following for an interesting salad:

carrots   red cabbage
squash   onions
cauliflower   sprouts
broccoli   spinach, raw
mushrooms   dark lettuce
fresh corn   avocado
raw peas   boiled eggs
bell pepper   cheese

Waldorf Salad

diced apples with skins	walnut, chopped
diced celery	mayonnaise

Combine all of the above and serve chilled. For low calorie salad, use mixture of half cottage cheese and yogurt in place of mayonnaise.

Winter Fruit Salad

Combine fruits which are plentiful in the winter such as oranges, apples, bananas, and pineapple. Serve plain or mix with yogurt topping made with plain yogurt and pure maple syrup.

SALAD DRESSINGS

Catsup

Chop 3 gallons ripe tomatoes. Liquify in blender. Put through a food mill to remove seeds. Blend in blender 2 large onions with 2 cups liquified tomatoes. Cook tomato juice and onion juice with 1 tablespoon salt and 1 tablespoon garlic powder until well done. Put in a cloth bag and drain one hour or more. Add 1 cup honey and 1 cup apple-cider vinegar. Cook 10 minutes and seal. Will make approximately 3 quarts of catsup.

Creamy Garlic

1 cup homemade buttermilk	½ tsp. sea salt
¼ tsp. garlic powder	1 tsp. parsley flakes
1 cup homemade mayonnaise	

Shake thoroughly and chill before serving. (Yogurt may be substituted for buttermilk.)

French Dressing

¾ cup safflower oil	½ tsp. sea salt
¼ cup lemon juice	¼ tsp. garlic powder
¼ tsp. paprika	½ cup homemade catsup or
¼ tsp. dry mustard	tomato sauce
½ tsp. celery seed	

Mix in the blender. Store in the refrigerator.

Health Dip

2 cups yogurt	¼ cup wheat germ
2 cups cottage cheese	¼ tsp. garlic powder
¼ cup sesame seeds	

Blend yogurt and cheese thoroughly. Add remaining ingredients. Chill and serve with raw cauliflower, carrots, celery, bell pepper and broccoli.

Italian Dressing

1 cup safflower oil	½ tsp. oregano leaves
¼ cup lemon juice	½ tsp. dry mustard
¼ cup apple-cider vinegar	½ tsp. paprika
½ tsp. sea salt	⅛ tsp. thyme
1 tsp. honey	2 cloves garlic, crushed

Shake all ingredients in tightly covered jar. Refrigerate.

Mayonnaise

1 egg	¼ tsp. paprika
½ tsp. salt	2 tbsp. lemon juice
½ tsp. dry mustard	1 cup safflower oil

Place the egg, seasonings, vinegar, lemon juice into the blender. Cover and blend. Remove feeder cap and pour in the oil in a steady stream. Store in the refrigerator.

Thousand Island Dressing

¼ cup finely chopped celery	1 cup mayonnaise
¼ cup finely chopped green pepper	¼ cup home-made catsup
¼ cup finely chopped green onion	2 hard-cooked eggs, finely chopped

Combine all ingredients, mix well. Store in refrigerator.

SNACKS AND DESSERTS

Banana Smoothie

2 cups milk	¼ cup honey
2 bananas, peeled and sliced	1 tsp. pure vanilla

Blend in the blender until frothy. (Bananas can be sliced and frozen in the freezer to make a milk-shake-type drink.)

Banana Crunch

Mix equal amounts of:

dried banana slices
carob-covered soy nuts
almonds

Soy nuts may be covered with carob by melting 1 cup carob chips, 1 tablespoon honey and 1 teaspoon water over low heat. Stir in soy nuts. Pour on waxed paper and allow to cool. After cooling, break into small pieces.

Basic White Frosting

   1 cup powdered coconut sugar (see p. 135)
   2 tbsp. softened butter
   4 tbsp. warm milk
 ½ tsp. pure vanilla
   2 tbsp. honey or pure maple syrup

Blend thoroughly and spread on top of cake or cookies.

Carob Chip Cookies

½ cup butter	½ tsp. sea salt
⅔ cup honey	1 tsp. soda
2 beaten eggs	1 cup carob chips, unsweetened
1 tsp. vanilla	1 cup chopped nuts
2½ cup whole-wheat flour	

Cream butter, add honey, eggs, and vanilla. Add dry ingredients. Mix in chips and nuts. Beat well. Drop by teaspoonful on cookie sheet. Press flat with fork. Bake at 350° for 10 minutes.

Carob Clusters

1 cup carob chips, unsweetened	1 tsp. water
3 tbsps. honey	1½ cups unsalted peanuts (may be half raisins)

Over low heat, melt carob, honey, and water. Stir in peanuts and raisins. Cool 10 minutes and drop by teaspoons onto cookie sheet covered with waxed paper. Chill to harden.

Carob Syrup

When your recipe calls for bitter or unsweetened chocolate, use 1 cup carob and 1 cup water blended together. Mix carob and water in a small saucepan. Bring to a boil, using low heat. Stir constantly. Cook for 5 minutes or until syrup is completely smooth. When the recipe calls for melted semi-sweet chocolate, use the above mixture plus ¼ cup honey and 1 to 2 tablespoons butter. Store this mixture covered in the refrigerator.

Carrot Cake

1 cup safflower oil	½ cup pineapple
3 eggs	½ cup raisins
¾ cup honey	1 tsp. cinnamon
¼ cup molasses	3 cups whole-wheat flour
2 cups carrots, grated	½ cup coconut

Beat oil, eggs, honey and molasses. Beat in rest of the ingredients. Bake in greased 9 x 13 pan at 350° for 45 minutes. Ice with Cream Cheese Frosting (next recipe).

Cream Cheese Frosting

Mix cream cheese, apple juice or honey and butter until smooth. Spread on top of cake.

Crisp Honey Cookies

½ cup butter	½ tsp. cinnamon
½ cup honey	¼ tsp. ground cloves
1¾ cup whole-wheat flour	1 tsp. soda

Cream butter and honey. Add dry ingredients. Chill one hour. Roll to ⅛ " thickness. Cut with cookie cutter. Bake at 350° for 8-10 minutes.

Frozen Banana Sticks

Cut banana in half and place on a stick. Roll the banana in yogurt and then in seeds or nuts. Freeze.

Fruit Delight

2 cups plain yogurt	1 cup blueberries or peaches
2 bananas, sliced	¼ cup orange juice concentrate
1 cup honey	

Stir these together and process in ice cream maker or use the freezer process with ice cream recipe.

Fruit Drink

1 cup strawberries
1 cup bananas
2 cups apple juice

Blend in the blender. Pour into tall glasses.

Fruit Juice Popsicles

Mix together equal amounts of orange juice, apple juice and cranberry juice. Freeze after molding.

Fruit Leather

Apricot—Pit apricots; do not peel. Put four or five halves in the blender. Use puree setting. Add one teaspoon honey to each cup of puree.

Line a cookie sheet with plastic wrap. Spread approximately 2 cups of puree almost to the edges. Leave a small amount of plastic wrap uncovered around the edges so it will be easy to remove. Put this on a table to dry in the hot sun. It will take approximately 6 to 8 hours to dry depending on the heat and humidity or place in 150° oven with door ajar until dried.

Peel the fruit off the plastic while the fruit is still warm. Roll the fruit leather in the plastic and store in a paper sack. This may be kept for some time.

Apple—Use 2 cups of puree for each cookie sheet. Sweeten to taste. Cinnamon may be added for variation. Do not use crisp, hard apples.

Peach—Peel, if desired. Use 2½ to 3 cups puree per sheet. Sweetening is optional. (If puree is too thin, the result will be fruit chips.)

Fruit Slush

Chill any fruit juice in the freezer until slightly frozen. Shake and serve.

Grandma's Raw Apple Cake

4 cups apples, chopped	1 tsp. sea salt
1 cup honey	½ tsp. cinnamon
2 tsp. vanilla	2 tsp. baking soda
2 eggs	2 cups whole-wheat flour
½ cup safflower oil	1 cup chopped walnuts

Mix the apples, honey and vanilla together and let stand for ½ hour. Put the eggs and oil into the apple mixture. Add salt, cinnamon, and baking soda. Add flour and walnuts. Mix together and bake 350° for 40 to 45 minutes. Turn oven off and let cake stay in another 5 minutes.

Honey Candy

¾ cup sesame seeds or slivered almonds	⅓ cup butter
	¼ cup honey

Butter 9 x 9-inch pan. Melt butter and honey in a heavy skillet. Cover for about 3 minutes. Cook over medium heat, stirring constantly, until mixture turns golden brown (about 2 to 4 minutes). Place sesame seeds in bottom of pan. Spread mixture in prepared pan while still hot. Cut into squares immediately with buttered knife. Cool. Yield, 36 squares.

Honey Popcorn Balls

1 cup honey	¼ cup water
1 tsp. vanilla	2 quarts of popcorn

Mix the honey and water. Put on high heat and stir until it boils. Change heat to medium and stir. Drop part of mixture into a cup of cold water. When it forms a ball, (235°) remove the pan from the heat. Add vanilla. Pour over popcorn and form balls. If desired, add ½ cube butter while cooking to make caramel corn.

Ice Cream

1 cup cream	¾ cup honey
2 cups fruit (your choice)	enough milk to make ½ gallon
3 eggs	

Blend evaporated milk, fruit, eggs and honey in the blender. Add enough milk to make ½ gallon. Process in an ice cream maker or freeze in a 9 x 13 pan in your freezer. After ice crystals have formed, remove from freezer. Beat with mixer. Return to freezer until set up.

Nature's Crunch

Mix equal amount of:

raisins	sunflower seeds
peanuts	dates, chopped
carob chips	

No-Bake Peanut Butter Cookies

3 cups rolled oats	¾ cup honey
½ cup milk	1 tsp. vanilla
½ cup peanut butter	1 cup nuts or may use crunchy peanut butter

Place oats in 350° oven to toast. In a pan mix milk, peanut butter, and honey and bring to a boil. Pour over oats. Add vanilla. Mix lightly. Let cool 5 minutes. Shape into balls. Roll in nuts or coconut.

Orange Julius

1 cup milk	1 cup water
¼ cup honey	10 ice cubes
1 cup orange juice concentrate	1 tsp. vanilla

Mix in the blender.

Peanut Brittle

1 cup honey
1 tbsp. butter
1 tsp. vanilla

1 tsp. soda
2 cups raw peanuts

Cook honey to hard crack stage, 300°. Remove from heat. Add butter, vanilla and soda. Pour in peanuts. Pour out on buttered cookie sheet. Break into pieces after cooling.

Peanut Butter Bars

1½ cups granola
1 cup powdered milk

1 cup peanut butter
½ cup honey

Press in a 9 x 9-inch pan. Chill and cut into bars.

Peanut Butter Candy

1 cup peanut butter
½ cup each raisins and dry powdered milk
¼ cup sesame seeds
¼ cup honey

Mix together, roll in one-inch balls, refrigerate.

Peanut Butter Clay

1 cup peanut butter (creamy)
½ cup honey

1 cup dry powdered milk

Mix peanut butter and honey together. Stir in dry powdered milk. Spend time playing with the children teaching them to use a rolling pin and cookie cutter.

Pecan Pie

¾ cup butter
4 eggs
3 tbsp. milk
¾ cup honey

1 tsp. vanilla
1 tbsp. wheat flour
1 cup pecans

Cream butter. Beat in eggs, honey and milk. Add remaining ingredients. Pour in whole-wheat pie shell. Bake for 30-40 minutes until knife comes out clean.

Popped Wheat

Soak wheat in cold water for 24 hours, changing the water once or twice during this time. Drain wheat and rinse. Let excess water drain off by placing on a towel. In a heavy skillet, heat oil to 350-400°. Place about ½ cup of wheat in a strainer and deep fry for about 1½ minutes.

An electric fry pan could be used. Put the wheat kernels directly in the oil and strain after frying. Drain on absorbent paper. Serve with salt as desired.

Powdered Coconut Sugar

Place unsweetened, dried coconut in blender. Process at medium speed until coconut is very fine. Store in sealed glass jar in refrigerator. Use in place of powdered sugar to sweeten donuts, cookies, small cakes and buns.

Pumpkin Pie

1½ cup pumpkin	½ tsp. sea salt
2 cups milk	1 tsp. cinnamon and nutmeg
½ to 1 cup honey	4 eggs, beaten
1 cup fresh cream	

Mix and heat all but eggs to boiling point. Remove from stove, add eggs. Pour mixture into two crusts baked 4 minutes. Bake at 350° for 45 minutes.

Strawberry Shortcake

⅓ cup honey	1 cup unbleached flour
¼ cup safflower oil	½ cup wheat germ
¼ tsp. sea salt	½ cup milk
1 tsp. vanilla	2 tsp. baking powder
1 egg	½ cup soy flour

Blend honey and oil. Add unbeaten egg and vanilla. Beat thoroughly. Mix dry ingredients together. Add to liquid mixture. Pour into greased loaf pan. Bake 35 minutes at 350°. Serve with fresh strawberries and whipped cream.

Yogurt Popsicle

2 cups yogurt	2 mashed bananas
1 tsp. vanilla	1 cup frozen orange juice concentrate

Mix together until smooth. Pour into molds. Freeze.

Zucchini Bread

	1 tsp. soda
1 cup safflower oil	1 tsp. cinnamon
1 cup honey	¼ tsp. baking powder
3 eggs	1 tsp. vanilla
3 cups whole-wheat flour	1 cup nuts (optional)
½ tsp. sea salt	2 cups zucchini

Combine oil and honey. Add to beaten eggs. Combine dry ingredients. Combine the two mixtures, adding grated zucchini. Bake at 350° for 40 minutes. Makes 2 loaves. Variations:

Banana Bread: 2 cups mashed ripe banana. Omit cinnamon and zucchini.

Pumpkin Bread: 2 cups pumpkin, ½ teaspoon cloves, allspice and ginger. Omit zucchini.

All of these may be cooked in a bundt pan at 300° for 1 hour and 25 minutes.

For additional recipes: send for *Eat Your Way to ... Health ... and Enjoy It!* by Johanna Hall, 1104 Hartwood Avenue, Virginia Beach, Virginia 23454.

Bibliography

Aikman, Lonnelle. *Nature's Healing Arts.* Washington, D.C.: National Society, 1977.

Albright, Nancy. *The Rodale Cookbook.* Emmaus: Rodale Press, Inc., 1973.

Anderson, Arthur W. *Bee Prepared With Honey.* Bountiful: Horizon Publishers, 1975.

Boie, Shirley A. *Herbs and How to Use Them.* Los Angeles: Boie Enterprises, 1978.

Bricklin, Mark. *The Practical Encyclopedia of Natural Healing.* Emmaus: Rodale Press, 1976.

Bricklin, Mark. *Rodale's Encyclopedia of Natural Home Remedies.* Emmaus: Rodale Press, 1982.

Brody, Jane. *Jane Brody's Nutrition Book.* New York: Bantam Books, 1981.

Cheraskin, E., M.D., D.M.D. and W. M. Ringsdorf, Jr., D.M.D., M.S. *Psycho-Dietetics.* New York: Bantam Books, 1974.

Clark, Linda. *Get Well Naturally.* New York: Arco Publishing Company, 1965.

Davis, Adelle. *Let's Eat Right to Keep Fit.* New York: Harcourt, Brace and Company, 1954.

Davis, Adelle. *Let's Get Well.* New York: Harcourt, Brace and Company, 1965.

Davis, Adelle. *Let's Have Healthy Children.* New York: Harcourt, Brace and Company, 1951.

Davis, Adelle. *Let's Stay Healthy.* Chicago: Signet Books, 1981.

Dienstbier, Sharon B., and Sybil D. Hendricks. *Natural Food Storage Bible.* Bountiful: Horizon Publishers, 1976.

Dickey, Esther. *Passport to Survival.* Salt Lake City: Bookcraft, Inc., 1969.

Dufty, William. *Sugar Blues.* Radner: Chilton Book Company, 1975.

"Fats. Are They Good or Bad For Us?" *Nutrition Now!* March 1980.

Ethington, Evelyn C. *Creative Wheat Cookery.* Bountiful: Horizon Publishers, 1975.

Feingold, Ben F. *Why Your Child Is Hyperactive.* New York: Random House, 1975.

Fryer, Lee and Dick Simmons. *Earth Foods.* Chicago: Follett Publishing Company, 1972.

Gerras, Charles. *The Complete Book of Vitamins.* Emmaus: Rodale Press, 1977.

Griffin, LaDean. *Is Any Sick Among You?* Provo: Bi-World, 1974.

Heinerman, John. *Science of Herbal Medicine.* Orem: Bi-World, 1979.

Hunter, Beatrice Trum. *The Natural Foods Primer.* New York: Simon and Schuster, 1972.

Hunter, Kathleen. *Health Foods and Herbs.* New York: Arc Books, Inc., 1963.

Kerschman, John D. *Nutrition Almanac.* New York: McGraw-Hill Book Company, 1973.

Kinderlehrer, Jane. *Confessions of a Sneaky Organic Cook.* Emmaus: Rodale Press, Inc., 1971.

Kloss, Jethro. *Back to Eden.* Santa Barbara: Woodbridge Press Publishing Company, 1939.

Lansky, Vicki. *The Taming of the Candy Monster.* New York: Bantam Books, 1978.

Larimore, Bertha B. *Sprouting For All Seasons.* Bountiful: Horizon Publishers, 1975.

Lesser, Michael, M.D. *Nutrition and Vitamin Therapy.* New York: Bantam Books, 1980.

Lust, John, N.D., D.B.M. *The Herb Book.* New York: Bantam Books, 1974.

Malstrom, Dr. Stan, N.D., M.T., *Own Your Own Body.* Orem: Fresh Mountain Air Publishing Company, 1977.

Marsh, Edward E. *How to be Healthy with Natural Foods.* New York: Gramercy Publishing Company, 1963.

Mayer, Dr. Jean and Jeanne Goldberg, R.D. "Most Important Nutrient: Water," *The News-Sentinel,* September 11, 1980, p. 2C.

McGrath, William R. *Common Herbs for Common Illnesses.* Provo: Nu Life Publishing, 1977.

Miller, Marjorie. *Health Foods.* New York: Falahad Books, 1971.

Null, Gary. *The New Vegetarian.* New York: Williams Morrow and Company, Inc., 1978.

Paulding, Linus. *Vitamin C, the Common Cold and the Flu.* New York: Berkley Books, 1970.

Reuben, David, M.D. *Everything You Always Wanted to Know About Nutrition.* New York: Simon and Schuster, 1978.

Reuben, David, M.D. *The Save Your Life Diet.* New York: Ballantine Books, 1975.

Reuben, David, M.D. and Barbara Reuben, M.S. *The Save Your Life High Fiber Cookbook.* New York: Random House, 1975.

Robertson, Laurel, Carol Flinders and Bronwen Godfrey. *Laurel's Kitchen.* New York: Nilgiri Press, 1976.

Rodale, J. I. *The Complete Book of Food and Nutrition.* Emmaus: Rodale Books, 1972.

Shute, Wilfred E. *Vitamin E for Ailing and Healthy Hearts.* New York: Pyramid House, 1969.

Smith, Lendon, M.D. *Feed Your Kids Right.* New York: McGraw-Hill Book Company, 1979.

Smith, Lendon, M.D. *Foods for Healthy Kids.* New York: Berkley Books, 1981.

Stevens, James Talmage. *Making the Best of Basics.* Salt Lake City: Penton Corporation, 1975.

"Sugar: The Facts Are More Sour Than Sweet," *Nutrition Now!,* March 1980, p. 1, 3.

Taub, Harold Jay. *The Health Food Shopper's Guide.* New York: A Dell Trade Paperback, 1982.

Whittlesey, Marietta. *Killer Salt.* New York: Bolder Books, 1977.

Classes corresponding with this book are taught by certified instructors. For additional information about these classes or seminars in your area write or call P.O. Box 8132, Holland, Michigan 49422 or (219) 493-1938.

Index